CONTE

INTRODUCTION

My greatest hope as I write this book is that it acts as a bridge between the belief systems you currently have regarding your health - and what is possible. I sometimes reflect on whether I wrote this book or this book chose me to write it....?

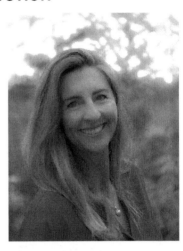

For as long as I can remember I have had an interest in health. I grew up in a house attached to a veterinary practice where I watched my dad treat animals of all descriptions. It wouldn't be unusual to have a horse on our drive waiting to be seen, or poorly animals in our kitchen by the Aga. The surgery itself held so much fascination for me. I would go in here as often as I could and even managed to "help" make appointments and answer the phone once I was a teenager. I listened to my dad prescribe medication or often just give advice and I watched in awe as he performed surgery, anaesthetise an animal and skilfully undertake whatever operation he was carrying out and then I watched the animals recover and go home. Sometimes, we all helped deliver puppies at 2am as no staff were there to help rub puppies until they squeaked, they were the most exciting nights. Those memories have stayed with me for decades. I grew up with a very medicalised view of the world. I saw drugs and surgery offer good solutions to every kind of ailment. However, things were about to change.

My mum was the perfect vet's wife, supportive and calm in all situations. She was a teacher by profession, yet maybe like me, had a secret passion for health and wellbeing. While I was still very young, she switched jobs. I know we think very little of career changes now but 40 years ago it was unusual. I watched my mum retrain as a Radionics practitioner and build a very successful practice. She developed a strong interest in homeopathy which rubbed off on my dad who decided to not only study it fully but to also teach and write books on the subject for vets. This led him to use homeopathy as an alternative to orthodox veterinary medicine for cases that did not respond to drugs. I witnessed first-hand amazing results for the animals he treated. I saw both approaches working in perfect synergy.

As my exposure to a holistic approach to health began when I was so young, I don't remember a time that I didn't have this belief. Animals can't speak, I know that is an obvious statement but what I mean is because they can't speak, I witnessed my dad ask questions at every consultation about every aspect of an animal's wellbeing. It was never about one symptom, it was always about making the correct diagnosis and then knowing the right treatment would follow.

What my dad saw each day, without even knowing it, was exactly the same as we are now witnessing in the human species. By domesticating animals, we remove them from their natural environment and this leads to chronic stress and diseases not previously seen. Chronic stress in animals and humans is a disease of our time and is requiring us to take a very different approach.

If you had a fish in a tank at home and the water was getting dirtier and dirtier and the fish looked sicker and sicker what would you do? I hope you'd clean the tank and improve the environment for the fish to live in. I doubt very much your first thought would be to put drugs into the water to help the fish. This is what we are seeing across all the animals we keep in captivity, their environment has changed and they are displaying sickness, yet we use drugs and surgery as a first approach, rather than look at the environment they find themselves in. Think about a caged tiger in a zoo, the way it paces up and down, has a poor appetite, develops fertility issues and joint pains. Would these things occur in the wild?? Are drugs the solution?

Many pets and captive animals develop health issues that would not have been seen in the wild and the analogy to man did not escape me. In fact it has screamed at me...again and again over many years, until I drew the only conclusion I could - we are now domesticated humans!

We are living caged lives.

So much of this book is about shining a light on the cage we have found ourselves in. I'll be looking at how we have deviated away from the life a "free, wild, natural" human would have lived - and seeing how far removed we now are from that.

Please don't think I am saying that we should all be living in caves and hunting and gathering still. What I am saying is, if that's what our bodies think we should be doing to fulfil our purpose as a human on this planet, then it gets a pretty big shock when day-to-day reality is so very different. Cars, offices, congestion, pollution, processed foods, lack of community and family all become a massive toxic load for us to carry.

I feel incredibly lucky to have grown up witnessing what I did, it formed thoughts that have grown over the years. I have a clear memory of overeating sweets as a child and discovering that if I went out for a walk when I felt "yucky" from that sugar overload, I quickly felt much better.

I learnt to enjoy feeling well and energised, as opposed to sluggish and ill and naturally migrated towards doing more of what made me feel good. I didn't know why or even what at first but my life's journey has been evolving ever since.

Much of what I have learnt is written in the pages of this book. Many things have become clearer to me as amazing leaders and teachers have crossed my path, as I have read different books and articles, seen research papers that prove or disprove theories. I have had a career in Chiropractic for more than 30 years and witnessed thousands of people improve their health. Satisfying...yes but I know my work isn't over yet. What I see on a daily basis are wonderful people struggling with solvable health issues - all they are missing is a bridge to enable them to cross from where they are now, to where they want to be.

My greatest hope for this book is that bridge - and once you get to the other side of your own belief systems, you can have freedom of choice on how to live a completely balanced, healthy lifestyle.

ACKNOWLEDGEMENTS

Firstly, I need to thank my parents for giving me a view of the world that was outside the conventional. It taught me to always be open-minded. Without that grounding, I may not have been on the journey I have.

Three amazing mentors have shaped my career and it would be remiss of me not to give them a huge amount of credit for keeping me on a path of discovery and opening my heart and mind to the power of the human body. Dr Simon King, you took a frustrated student and showed me the power of the human body to heal when interference is removed.

Dr Neil Davies, knowing you for the last 20 years has been an absolute privilege, from the first moment I heard you speak in a lecture theatre in Bournemouth, I knew you had a system and protocol that I wanted to master. Through learning NIP and working with babies and children, I have had the most rewarding career and know that I have positively impacted lives. You are one of the world's geniuses and what you have brought to the chiropractic profession is nothing short of a legacy.

Dr James Chestnut, you turned the light on for me in Wellness care. So much of what I already believed and knew, you condensed into the study of human health and wellbeing. You were the inspiration for me to write the Complete Lifestyle Guides and educate my community. You started me on a journey to change my life, my family's life and so many others. Thank you.

My deepest level of love and gratitude goes to my children and my husband, these amazing humans have lived every aspect of the Complete Lifestyle journey with me, from experimental foods and drinks (of very dubious colour), to supporting my workshops and monthly health plans. Feeding me and yourselves when I have been working on this book for many hours each day. Unconditionally believing in me and this mission to help others. For taking the road lesstravelled with me and working to make healthier choices each day even when your friends thought you were a bit crazy!

Watching the children struggle to defend their beliefs and trying to educate others both broke my heart and inspired me in equal measures. I know how hard it can be to help others see what you see. They never gave up, for that my gorgeous, grown-up babies, I love you so much.

I hope I have taught you that you have control of your own life, you can change anything you set your mind to.

This book has always been in me, it is filled with information I share on a daily basis. It is a description of the lifestyle we live and a deep look into the belief systems we run with.

Thank-you to every person that has ever listened to my advice, to every person that has changed their lives because of something I said or helped with. Thank-you also to the people that haven't wanted to hear what I have had to say, you inspire me to find another way to deliver my message.

Thank-you to my dad, John Saxton for help on edits for each and every chapter and to Helen Nash for finally pulling this together so it reads like a book. You are both so instrumental in this book being published, thank you.

My harshest critic, my greatest supporter, my soul mate, my best friend, my amazing husband Nigel. I know if I can get you to drink water and live this lifestyle, I can get anyone to! Thank-you for being my toughest nut to crack! I love you. X

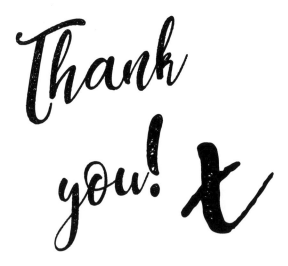

PREFACE

This book aims to introduce you to ideas about health and wellness, many of which will challenge the very core of your belief systems. It may initially be difficult to accept some of the ideas but if it can be read with an open mind, it will soon be possible to appreciate the sense behind what is suggested.

This is above all a self-help book, born out of my own study and experience, to enable you to understand how you, as an individual, can get yourself back to health and enjoy both a better quality and quantity of life.

In many ways, our phobias about getting old are worries about infirmity. It is not so much the thought of getting old that sends us into a flat spin as the thought of not being able to do the things we love, whatever that might be. The thought of not being independent terrifies us all.

I am sure that, like me, you love having energy and vitality and living each day pain-free with a smile on your face; that to me is living. In a word, wellness is what we all dream of but so often struggle to achieve. We should not blame ourselves completely as the information we receive is often extremely confusing and conflicting. However, if we keep listening to corporations, keep paying attention to adverts and celebrity endorsements, we will continue to fall into the same health traps over and over again.

All change requires a will and everyone has to find their own driving force. I have an amazing family that I want to be around for as long as I possibly can, I want to be a fit and healthy grandmother and possibly great-grandmother, too, Equally importantly, I want to be the best role model I can possibly be to encourage them to ensure their own good health . That is the driving force that leads my health decisions on a daily basis, and no doubt you will have your own incentives. At this point I must admit, I am no angel. I love treats and most days you can find me with a glass of wine in my hand as I cook dinner. However, I also make fresh juice daily, or have a nutrient-packed smoothie, I eat raw foods whenever possible, source only grass-fed meats and exercise daily. If that sounds like too much of an effort, you will be pleasantly surprised when you start on the journey that gets you the rewards of creating your own good health.

To get the best out of this book, you need to understand your present beliefs about health or maybe it would be better to ask you to think about how you view sickness. I'll make an educated guess at this point that you sit in one of two camps - either you believe that germs are the cause of disease, that they are invasive and random, are the cause of illness and the best approach is to manage symptoms and attack the germ with medication. Or, you believe that health is an inside job, that our own health is determined by the health of our own cells.

That the human body is programmed for health and if sickness is present then it is a response to a change in the environment that was keeping us balanced and healthy.

It is also just worth glancing at the epidemic proportions of chronic illness all around us and deciding if you believe these modern day diseases, such as arthritis, asthma, heart disease, cancer and diabetes etc are caused by our lifestyle or by our genetic makeup. Let us first go back to the germ theory...

Two gentlemen battled these theories out in the nineteenth century when Louis Pasteur and Antoine Bechamp had these two very opposing views. The germ theory VS the cellular theory. For those interested in the science behind each of these theories, a short internet search will provide much food for thought and solid information to build your views on.

I believe there are a number of reasons why the germ theory became so popular a century or more ago. There was a mechanistic view of the world, it was how people were explaining things and it was the model used when new things were discovered. It was easy to sell ideas to the public that fitted that model.

Couple that with the human trait of avoiding personal responsibility and the idea of germs invading us at will and it being completely out of our control fitted very nicely with a blame culture (we are not that different today!) Finally, there was a commercial gain to be made from the germ theory. As people took on the idea they were under attack, they then needed to be "rescued" and that opened the door for drug development, treatment protocols and the need to be "treated" to get rid of the disease. As far as I can see, our attitudes are basically the same today.

The reality is far different and was voiced, proven and sadly quashed hundreds of years ago, only to rise again, as the truth so often does. Bacteria do not invade us as often as we think, most are there all the time, the health of our own cells dictates whether they can get a hold and become pathogenic (cause sickness) or not. Health, or the lack of it, is an inside job! If you have healthy cells, you will have healthy organs, healthy body systems and everything will work in balance. Exactly as it is programmed to do.

"Disease is born of us and in us"

Bechamp

"We should not ask what sort of disease does this person have, but rather what sort of person has this disease"

Paracelsus

Backing the wrong horse has been done many times in history, this dominance of germ theory was in many ways a very costly mistake and has led to the pharmaceutical industry as we know it today and a medical profession with a paradigm that is rigid and strongly defensive of the germ theory. This makes crossing a path to wellness very hard and yet still the awakening consciousness to health is rising up.

Pasteur himself recounted in his private journal, writing the famous words which were revealed many decades after his death "It is not the germ that causes disease but the terrain in which the germ is found".

The rest of this book is based on the cellular theory because for me this is the truth behind our survival as a species. The theory is simple and applying the rules will deliver excellent health outcomes.

CHAPTER 1

The Iceberg - We Are Programmed for Health

If you cut your finger it heals, if you are cold you shiver, if you are hot you sweat, when you are invaded by pathogens your body temperature rises. You balance hormones, digest food, eliminate waste, think and move. You have a heart that beats over 80,000 times a day, every day of your life and lungs that deliver oxygen to every cell in your body every moment of your life.

The definition of health is quite simply -

THE BALANCE IN THE FUNCTION OF THE CELLS IN OUR BODIES

We have over 75 trillion cells and each one knows EXACTLY what to do when. How do they know that?? Quite simply, they are programmed that way. Can you imagine the chaos in your body if that statement was not true. If cells behaved randomly, sometimes functioning sometimes not. If they died off and weren't replaced. If they failed to perform their designated action. We simply would not function as human beings.

Our entire development from the coming together of two cells at conception is ingeniously orchestrated to create the miracle that is the human body. It is structured, designated, organised and duplicable. Like every other animal and plant on this planet, our cells know exactly what to do and when. If this was not a basic truth, we may survive one generation but we could not reproduce and therefore our species would die.

When there is a lack of balance in the cells of our bodies this creates the symptoms of sickness.

We know that a lack of balance does not create health and does not lead to a strong, thriving species. We are all aware that we are seeing pandemic levels of chronic ill health. Could it be possible that there is some advantage to chronic illness? Some benefit to us as individuals and us as a species trying to survive here on planet earth.

I think an analogy will help you understand the answer, and explain the title of this book Imagine you are a healthy person trapped on an iceberg, you have no equipment with you and only a few pieces of clothing. The outside temperature is dropping and you cannot get off the iceberg. At this point your body is going to be doing some extremely clever things, the single aim being to keep you alive. It will make you shiver, it will slow down all bodily functions that do not serve you at that time, like digestion, immune function and elimination, it will divert blood from your extremities to your heart and brain.

All these actions will happen automatically, without your intervention, because that is how you are programmed to respond. Your body is in survival mode now. As the hours tick by your physiology will continue to adapt, finally only keeping the minimum number of systems still functioning. It will sacrifice damaged toes, ears, nose and fingers if necessary.

It will slow all movement, depress respiration and slow the heart beat.

Your body is quite simply trying to keep you alive long enough for you to Get Off Your Iceberg!

Remember you were perfectly well when you got on the iceberg.

Not one symptom is random or incorrect, it is perfect.

Are you out of balance? Yes!

Are you feeling unwell? Yes!

Is it an incorrect response or is the body an absolute genius and you were the cause of the problem. After all you got on the iceberg in the first place.

To be well again you quite simply have to get off the iceberg. If you get off at the first sign of cold you will warm up quickly and have no ill effects from your temporary encounter with extreme cold. However if you ignore all the warning signs and symptoms that your body is out of balance, it is suffering and uncomfortable and if you continue to stay on the iceberg what will happen is that your body's adaptive ability can only keep you alive to a certain point. After that, the adaptation required becomes too much and your body can no longer function. From that extreme point you can no longer recover. Even interventions designed to save you cannot help and get enough cells functioning again to bring your body back to life.

We each have our own icebergs, we all sit on them observing symptoms appearing and using a sticking plaster approach to make that symptom go away. If we could learn to get off our icebergs, to change our environment our bodies would instantly revert back to functioning the way they are designed to - in perfect balance.

Before considering what actually changes our environment and how we can hypothetically get off our icebergs, think of a health scale for yourself. If zero is dead and 100% is perfect health, where would you honestly place yourself on that scale?

Think about some of the systems in your body and if you have any symptoms in them.

Do you have great energy?

Do you sleep well?

Do you have clarity of thought?

Do you have steady moods?

Do you have a strong immune system?

Do you have a healthy respiratory system?

Do you have a healthy cardiac system?

Do you have great movement and joints free of pain?

Do you have clear bright skin?

Do you have a good digestive system?

If you answered 'no' to any of the above or they triggered in you a reminder that you have things like low energy, poor sleep, dry skin, bloating or struggle with asthma or arthritis etc, then the rest of this book will change your life and you can see HOW to get off your iceberg and achieve the things shown above.

Your environment is your iceberg. Your environment will be either adding to the stress load on your body and causing it to adapt and show signs of sickness or it may be perfect for your body and you will exhibit great health and live symptom-free.

As long as you are alive, you can change, you can start to move up your own scale of health. Each and every day you can CHOOSE to do things that put you further and further up that scale and move you closer and closer towards balance. Call it the success curve of health.

The principle behind health is SO simple but the daily practise of it can be a little more challenging. Remember, if you can find a particular reason to be healthy rather than just a vague desire, then you will work at it more easily, so think now about what your reason would be.

CHAPTER 2

The Cause

If you can see that cellular balance in your body results in great health, then understanding what pushes us out of balance will help you take the first steps towards becoming healthier. Luckily, there are only two things that cause us to move out of cellular balance -

TOXICITY and DEFICIENCY

If we take a look at deficiency first, we can start to understand that this is when the body needs something and it is not being provided. This is a little like making a cake and not having eggs, you may create something but it will not be like the recipe you set out to make. In fact, you may choose just not to make the cake at all, once you find there are no eggs.

Either response at a cellular level will move you down the scale of health. So a top rule is to supply enough of everything the body needs to be well. This is such an important principle that you will meet it again and again as we explore how to create sufficiency in all the body needs.

The second cause is toxicity. This is a massive problem in the modern world; from the air we breathe, the water we drink, the food we eat, the products we use on our skin, the medication we take and so much more. Improving your knowledge on toxins and being determined to eliminate them from your lifestyle will result in a staggering improvement in your health. These two causes of cellular imbalance Deficiency and Toxicity occur in three areas. Each area should be considered when health goals are trying to be reached.

Giving the body a period of time when you can be both sufficient and toxin-free in all three areas results in a regaining of balance within the body and improved health. It is hard to emphasise the importance of that last sentence enough, it is viewed as the secret of true health. Because it is so important please read it again so you can digest the full meaning of it.

"The two causes of cellular imbalance Deficiency and Toxicity occur in three areas. Each must be addressed and true health can only return once you have established sufficiency and been toxin-free in all three areas for a period of time."

These three areas are: how we move, what we eat and what we think.

If you can learn how to eat, move and think in a different way, you will find yourself moving up the success curve of health.

This is a process, it will take you time to address and correct all these areas, however with a kick-start programme and the support and information in this book, you will have the tools you need to achieve your health goal.

Deprivation and sacrifice are poor lifestyle choices and almost certainly doomed to fail. How many times have you been on a diet only to lose weight and regain it just weeks later? Many people do this for decades of their lives, they try soup diets, calorie- controlled diets, water diets, brown rice diets, juice diets, all with no long-term success. Just a feeling of deprivation and the only thing that made the days on those "diets" bearable was the thought that they would end. Good health does not end, you want to choose a lifestyle that sustains it, and one that never leaves you with a feeling of sacrifice and deprivation. Humans, in fact all creatures, do not thrive in an environment of deprivation and we merely manage to survive when we find ourselves in that situation.

Success comes to those that can make a shift in their belief about health and truly understand the new choices they make. When that happens all decisions become easy.

For example, if you were offered a piece of chocolate knowing it had arsenic on it, would you take it? No, of course not because you know and believe that it would kill you. And you would be right! You have knowledge and evidence that arsenic kills you so you know to turn away from that option. If you can open your mind and consider changing your belief system about other things too, you can discover an amazing power that is borne out of knowledge.

Understanding some of the pitfalls you fall into and learning never to fall into them again is what this book is about. Learning the outline rules and living within them, you can rediscover a body that is healthy, a mind that is happy and a life that is fulfilled. That is the gift of good health.

Wellness is a wonderful concept and the goal we should all aim for. There is no diet or restrictive plan to govern every day, just a commitment to decide each day to make choices that will make and keep you well.

Many people already have diagnosed illnesses or may suffer an acute emergency that requires medical care. Modern medicine is amazing, it saves lives, prolongs lives and in many cases alleviates suffering, however, all medicine involves a pay-off between relieving a symptom and the toxic effects of the drugs prescribed. There is no drug that does not have a side effect, so deciding when and where to use drugs and surgery is a very important question. Can drugs and surgery create complete health? Or is it more likely that they merely relieve symptoms?

Imagine your body is a house and the medical profession is the fire brigade. If a fire broke out in your house who would you call? The obvious answer is the fire brigade. When they arrive at your house they would get out the tools of their trade, axes and fire hoses (drugs and surgery), they would smash down your doors and walls and spray water everywhere and if you were really lucky they would save your house. But when you return to your house and look around at the shell that remains, at the damage caused to save the main structure would your first thought be to call back the fire brigade to restore the health of your house?

Here is a lightbulb moment for many people as they can see the amazing benefit of an emergency-based system to save your life and the stupidity of using that emergency system to restore health?

It will never work! For all the miracles that emergency medicine performs, creating health is not one of them. You will never be healthier for having your tonsils out or taking painkillers but you will be saved from symptoms and, in the most severe cases of ill-health, medicine saves many lives. BUT to create health - or in the analogy restore the house - you need different people, you need builders, joiners, painters and decorators. They come with completely different tools and perform completely different functions but each group looks impotent in each other's role. A hammer and nails will never save your house but equally an axe and fire hose will never restore its structure.

Make sure you understand this difference, invest in the health of your house and you may never need the fire brigade. You will invest time and money in the use of joiners and decorators and keep a close eye on general continual maintenance of your house, noticing early if some extra work needs to be done. This way you do not live in fear of a fire, instead you trust in the strong safe state of your home. This is simultaneously a revolutionary and yet simple approach to great health.

Medicine looks at naming disease and treating it. Over the years it has just got better and better at naming and treating disease but it has never tried to create health as its priority. Doctors do not study health and how to create it; they study disease and how to treat it.

If you can understand that pills may make you feel better, but they will never make your cells function better, then you will have taken a massive step towards changing deeply ingrained beliefs about health. Sadly, drugs are toxic to our cells and actually decrease cell function. Even though they make you feel better, you get chronically sicker and sicker while on them.

Millions of pills are consumed every day in the western world and that number is increasing every year. These are prescribed pills treating chronic, preventable illnesses. Prescription drugs are currently responsible for more deaths per year than illegal drugs. There are almost 800,000 deaths in the western world from conventional medical mistakes each year. (That's the equivalent of seven jumbo jet crashes every day for the entire year!) more than 100,000 are from prescription drugs alone. Alarmingly, this number rises every year.

The American Medical Association estimates that almost 300 people die every day from prescription drug use (iatrogenic illness) alone in the USA. These are preventable deaths.

It is worth considering that for the last 60 years there have been more medical doctors, more nurses, more drugs, more hospitals and more money spent per person in the UK and most other industrialised nations, yet every year the rates of chronic sickness and preventable death increases.

Do you think it is possible people are looking for the answers in the wrong place or maybe asking the wrong questions?

CHAPTER 3

The Stress Response

The stress response is a survival response otherwise known as the flight or fight response. The changes that occur in our bodies when we perceive a stressor are designed to save our lives by giving us the ability to either fight or run away. Every time you think of a stressor, imagine that a tiger is chasing you, as no matter what caused the stress your body reacts exactly as if a tiger was chasing you. Understanding the stress response becomes much easier once this key point is understood; your body cannot differentiate between a tiger and a stressful phone call, a toxic meal or sitting too long. A stress is a stress as far as the body is concerned and it launches into a predetermined set of responses EVERY TIME it comes under stress.

Our biochemical and physiological stress response is designed for a fast reaction and to be over in a few minutes - the logic being we would either outrun the tiger or be eaten! Unfortunately for us, modern-day living is filled with low-grade, ongoing stressors and not so many tigers! The survival mechanism of the stress response, that is embedded in our blueprint, is designed to save us in an emergency and it is now being forced to play a very different role and it is a role with serious consequences.

All chronic illnesses can be attributed to the stress response. To help you understand that more clearly, study the chart below and begin to see the links for yourself in the programmed physiology of the body and then the effects on the body when the stress is sustained.

Now think back for a moment to when you were sitting on the iceberg - as you were sitting there freezing on your iceberg, very intelligently your blood was diverted away from all your extremities, your heart rate slowed, your breathing became laboured, your core temperature dropped. If at that moment you were magically taken off the iceberg, dropped into a GP's clinic and checked over, your vital statistics would not look great. You would be told how ill you are. You would be diagnosed and treated for each individual symptom. Imagine you did not tell the Doctor that you had been in the cold for hours, imagine you just listed your symptoms. What conclusion do you think they would draw?

Chronic ill health is like this, we are not honest about our own stress load, our own iceberg.

We fail to disclose the areas of our lives that are out of balance. Maybe we do this because we just did not know there was a link and maybe we are not asked this because the doctor's paradigm to treat sickness is far removed from the paradigm to find a root cause and create health. Lifestyle questions are rarely put at the front of any case history form.

To take another example, imagine you have just been for a run, your body's physiology is altered to support you through that activity. Your physiology is changed, your blood pressure is high, your pulse rate is up, your heart rate is up, you are sweating. Are you ill? If you took just those symptoms and never asked what you have just been doing, you would never know that running was the cause. You would see bodily function off balance and deem that person to be sick.

If you mix these stories around, you will understand that the body is adapting perfectly to the environment it is in at that time and you will appreciate just how clever your body is,bordering on genius, it knows EXACTLY what to do and when. It ALWAYS responds appropriately. If we could improve the quality of questions we ask when assessing lifestyle and ask the questions that help identify where the stress load is high and how it can be decreased, we would have a phenomenal opportunity to help people "get off their icebergs" and regain balance in their bodies and therefore watch health improve.

The miracle of our body's physiology is that it is changeable and instantly responsive. If you run your heart rate will rise, it must rise, your body needs oxygen faster than when you are at rest. Your body will NEVER make a change unless it is absolutely necessary at that moment for your best health outcome and ultimate survival. Medicating you for an increased heart rate and increased blood pressure at that moment would be ludicrous and cause all sorts of secondary problems.

If a foot is amputated for frost bite but the patient is left out in the cold, all that is achieved is the resolution of one symptom, the cause remains and as sure as night follows day another symptom will pop up, like a warning sign. The body is desperately trying to say that it needs to be in a different, healthier environment. Then, and only then, can it regain balance and be healthy. In the summary below the commonest physiological responses to stress are discussed and the response is explained, shedding light on why it occurs and how that helps us when we are under stress. Your body will not compromise on its response, it never gives half a response or forgets to respond. It will ensure it happens every time you are stressed about anything.

Increased Heart Rate

In the stress response, your body presumes you will need to run or fight; for that you require oxygen and nutrients in all the tissues of your body so your heart rate MUST rise to deliver on that.

Increased Blood Pressure

To get blood around your body faster, the pressure at which it leaves your heart will increase, a rise in blood pressure is a temporary consequence if your body is to deliver on this response.

Increased Blood Cholesterol

Cholesterol and fat are like rocket fuel for energy, to give you the best chance to run or fight with power and energy. It must be released into your bloodstream so it can be distributed around the body and utilised for energy. An increase in blood cholesterol levels will be detected as the body delivers on this need.

Increased Blood Clotting Factors

These pour into the bloodstream when you are under stress, the body is preparing for a potential wound and will need clotting factors present at the site of injury fast if it is to help you survive. Clotting factors will be increased in your blood to deliver on this need.

Increased Blood Glucose Levels

Glucose levels in our blood are constantly being balanced. Glucose is the human body's primary source of fuel. What is not used is stored in our muscles and liver and enough is stored for 24hours at any one time. When we are under stress we release glucose into our blood stream for energy. We need fuel and lots of it, running or fighting are high cost energy activities and we need to be ready for action. High blood glucose levels will be found in anyone exhibiting a stress response, we must do this to deliver more energy when the body needs it.

Increased Blood Lipid Levels

Pouring fats into our bloodstream is a really smart response when you need fuel for energy, blood test someone in this response and you will see increased lipid levels in the blood.

Insulin Resistance

Insulin production is temporarily switched off to ensure there is very little in our bloodstream as we need to keep blood glucose levels high for energy to run or fight. Without this, all the glucose we poured into the bloodstream for fuel would instantly be "neutralised" by the insulin in the bloodstream and placed back in storage. In the stress response, the pancreas appears non-responsive to high glucose levels, this is essential if the body is to maintain high glucose levels for energy.

Decreased Cellular Immunity

The immune system is one of the most energy-hungry systems in our bodies, when we are trying to fight or run as a response to stress, the immune response is turned off to save energy. This is intended to be only a short-term measure. However, in chronic stress this is happening for days, weeks and years and the consequences are severe - although to deliver more energy the body is still making a smart choice in response to stress.

Mental Capacity

Some very interesting things happen in our nervous systems and thought patterns in response to stress. We get extremely heightened perception of our immediate environment, with little attention to anything happening around us. We put a complete halt on memory and recollection, we enter into the fear response and suppress all production of serotonin - the happy hormone. We are on edge, alert, distracted from anything other than our current need to escape and we are anything but happy!

Increased Breakdown of Muscle and Connective Tissue

This happens in order to release minerals into the bloodstream and it also happens as a response to priming the tissues for action. We have an increased sensitivity to touch and pain and all cellular regeneration within the musculoskeletal system is stopped. This is not the time to concentrate on growth and repair, this is survival mode.

Increased Anabolic Steroids in our Bloodstream

These hormones help us to be stronger when strength is needed but they can also be very destructive if they do not disappear quickly from our blood system once the danger has passed. As a response to danger they are fabulous, if they linger they will weaken tissue and destroy bone.

- An increased in the stress hormones; adrenalin, nor-adrenalin & cortisol as soon as these are released into the blood stream **all** the following responses occur

- Increased heart rate
- Increased blood pressure
- Increased blood cholesterol levels
- Increased clotting factors

What do these lead to?

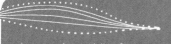

- Increased sensitivity of sensory systems, including those for pain
- Increased breakdown of muscle and connective tissue
- Decreased anabolic hormones
- Bone loss

What do these lead to?

- Increased blood glucose levels
- Increased blood lipid levels
- Insulin resistance

What do these lead to?

- Increased sensitivity of sensory systems, including those for pain
- Increased breakdown of muscle and connective tissue
- Decreased anabolic hormones
- Bone loss

What do these lead to?

- Decreased celluar immunity

What do these lead to?

Heart disease and strokes Diabetes & Obesity Muscle cramps, joint pain, arthritis, osteoporosis Depression, anxiety, ADHD Colds, flus and cancers

These responses all play an important role in surviving a stressful encounter, they are all appropriate, strategic and essential for our survival. However, the entire stress response is built on the premise that it is a fast, short-term response. Nothing in its design is helpful long term.Modern day living is putting our bodies into a continuous cycle of response to stress. The three stress categories are what we eat, how we move and what we think.

Add all these together and it is easy to understand why we get into this reactive stress response so many times a day.

The consequences are around us all, chronic illness in western society is at epidemic proportions, you may even be in that cycle yourself. Metabolic Syndrome X is the name given to the set of symptoms that appear when people are under chronic stress - high blood pressure, increased cholesterol levels, insulin resistance, poor memory, osteoporosis, joint degeneration among others. What started as a normal physiological response to save our lives in an emergency is being triggered inappropriately and is quite simply the cause of more deaths than any specific disease currently seen in our society.

By putting some of the normal responses together, it is easy to appreciate how they would present as medical findings as opposed to the normal physiological responses that they are.

Increased heart rate
Increased blood pressure
Increased blood cholesterol levels
Increased clotting factors
HEART DISEASE AND STROKES

Increased blood glucose levels
Increased blood lipid levels
Insulin resistance
DIABETES AND OBESITY

Decreased celluar immunity
COLDS, FLUS AND CANCERS

Increased feelings of stress, fear, anxiety and depression
Decreased short-term memory, ability to concentrate, and learn new material
Decreased serotonin; increased noradrenalin levels
DEPRESSION, ANXIETY, ADHD

Increased sensitivity of sensory systems, including those for pain
Increased breakdown of muscle and connective tissue
Decreased anabolic hormones
Bone loss
MUSCLE CRAMPS, JOINT PAIN, ARTHRITIS, OSTEOPOROSIS

The great news is that we have the power to prevent any and all of these conditions and many others. It comes down to the simple question if we can detect and control individual stress responses, we will have the power to prevent all of these illnesses.

Remember what health is – it is the BALANCE in the function of all the cells in the body.

A balanced body by definition is not stressed.

What causes stress – **TOXICITY and DEFICIENCY** in one or more of the three areas, how we **EAT, MOVE and THINK**

Address toxicity and deficiency in how we eat and we will be well.

Address toxicity and deficiency in how we move and we will be well.

Address toxicity and deficiency in how we think and we will be well.

Diseases can be prevented by removing the stressors. The next few chapters are going to cover some key stressors that will need to be addressed in order to achieve health. Bear in mind that it is no good being really good in one area and using that as an excuse to be out of balance in another. Exercising regularly and yet eating a poor diet will not deliver great health results. Likewise you may be someone who carries the worries of the world in their heads and yet tries really hard with your diet and exercise plans, again this will fall short when you are looking for the best health outcomes. If you have a diagnosed illness right now, I would encourage you to be vigilant in your approach and work on every sector simultaneously. You have a lot to gain, you have slipped a long way down the health slope and need to regain a lot of ground. Find your motivator, find your reason to fight and then get to work.

If you are working to prevent yourself getting on this slippery path to ill-health then you need to apply all the same rules, you just have a little more time on your side.

CHAPTER 4

Allergenic, Acidic and Addictive Foods

It is necessary at this point to consider the bowels - where millions of bacteria live. These help you digest all your food and are 75 per cent responsible for the functioning of the immune response. Known collectively as bowel (or gut) flora they are vital to the body's wellbeing.

Gut Flora

As long as the balance of the gut flora is correct, the bacteria are our friends but if that balance is upset, then they become the enemy within!

We all have approximately 1kg of this flora in our bowels; it lines the membranous cells of the bowel wall and, performs an invaluable task creating the link between digestion and immunity. We have a symbiotic relationship with these bacteria. What we need, they need; when we are well, they are well; when they function poorly, so do we. You will most likely have heard of Candida, this is a very common problem where the yeast-based bacteria proliferate due to our high sugar diets, at the cost of other bacteria - and this upsets the balance. Many symptoms appear when this balance is upset, they are sometimes just small and irritating and other times life-threatening. It is not uncommon these days to be trying to improve bowel health, sometimes this requires a very strict regime and at other times just a few small tweaks to diet and the use of a high-quality probiotic are enough to see dramatic changes in health.

As with so many things, we are responsible for the imbalance that develops; nature knows exactly what it is doing and without interferences would continue to work very effectively. But our personal stress load potentially upsets this balance and our health suffers.

Imbalance in the bowel flora has been linked to all the following conditions:

The general signs include pain, infection, fatigue and body malfunctions such as adrenal/thyroid failure, indigestion, diarrhoea, food cravings, intestinal pain, depression, hyperactivity, antisocial behaviour, asthma, haemorrhoids, colds, flu, respiratory problems, endometriosis, dry skin, itching, thrush, receding gums, nail fungus, dizziness, joint pain, bad breath, ulcers, colitis, heartburn, dry mouth, PMS, menstrual problems, irritability, puffy eyes, low sex drive, skin rash, hives, lupus, mood swings, allergies, hormonal imbalance, vaginal yeast infection, cysts, tumours, rheumatoid arthritis, numbness, hayfever, acne, gas/bloating, bowel stasis, low blood sugar, hiatal hernia, headaches, lethargy, laziness, insomnia, suicidal tendencies, coldness/shakiness, over/underweight conditions, chemical sensitivity, poor memory, muscle aches, burning eyes, multiple sclerosis, malabsorption, and bladder infections.

There are dozens of types of bacteria inside us and when present in perfect amounts, do us nothing but good, but some of the bacteria can survive in what would be considered a hostile environment and these will thrive in that situation at the expense of the other bacteria that need more exact conditions to perform their jobs. The balance is delicate and precise.

Just as we have a perfect body temperature, we also have a perfect internal pH, this is a measure of our internal acidity and alkalinity. With our body temperature, we run into some huge problems with basic survival outside a relatively narrow acceptable range. Our internal acid/alkaline level must also be maintained within a very small range or the body goes into a buffering response that corrects the balance. However, the cost of that response can sometimes be very high. Our normal pH is neutral to slightly alkaline; we do not thrive in an acid environment. Except for the acid in our stomach, which has some very specialised cells to deal with the pH level, there is no area of the body that functions happily in an acid environment. Some of our bowel bacteria however have found a way to survive the acid environment and do thrive. These have been popularly termed "bad" bacteria and they thrive at the expense of the "good" bacteria. Once the balance is lost we develop symptoms, many of which can be found on the list above.

For anyone who has ever taken antibiotics the chances are their bowel bacteria were wiped out. Just as their name suggests these drugs are anti- bacterial and that means the good bacteria in the bowels, as well as any bacteria attacking the body. The irony here is that by wiping out the bowel flora, three quarters of the immune function is compromised, thereby increasing the reliance on antibiotics to fight even the most minor infections. This is a very common presentation especially in children.

There is also the mounting concern regarding antibiotic resistance, this is a very real danger. It has been caused by over-prescribing antibiotics and the sheer resilience of bacteria. As they mutate and get stronger, our bodies get weaker due to lowered immune response and the antibiotics that were once effective are no longer. Mankind is faced with developing strains of superbugs and the real possibility of having no defence against them medically. In just a few years, there is every chance we will see epidemics of superbugs and be defenceless, unless of course we can call on our own "healthy" immune systems to respond to the challenge unhindered and do what it is programmed to do; fight infection.

There is one more part of the puzzle to look at before we can delve into what exactly makes our bowel unhealthy and that is a syndrome called the 'leaky gut syndrome'.

There is a time in our lives when this is beneficial and a time when it can make us very ill, When we were new born, we needed to develop our own immune systems. When we received the large molecule antibodies from our mother's breast milk it passed through our digestive system and ended up in our lower bowel. From here it passed into our blood stream through holes in our bowel wall. It was only when these molecules had passed into our blood stream that we had a defence against many pathogens. This is a passive form of immune defence, designed to bridge a gap between being a defenceless newborn and a human with a robust immune system. The antibodies we receive from our mothers give us temporary protection while the immune system develops its active immunity to the world around us.

Unfortunately, as the holes are there and they are big enough to let a large molecule through, other things are also allowed to pass through, too. This is one of the problems with cows' milk protein molecules, they are very large and foreign to us as newborns. They are ingested through formula milk and pass through the upper digestive system and into the bowel, from there they will pass through the holes in the bowel wall and straight into the bloodstream. Large protein molecules that are foreign and in our bloodstream will cause an immune response. It is 'battle stations' as all systems come into play to destroy the foreign body! This early exposure and the immune response that is launched is now known to cause not only dairy intolerance but also set the stage for autoimmune diseases later in life. This is a perfect example of a system that was so perfectly designed and yet through man's intervention has become compromised and altered and disease can be the result.

This leaky gut syndrome can also affect us later in life . When it appears in our adult life it is caused by an unhealthy bowel lining that becomes penetrable and once again allows access to the bloodstream directly. Again the passage of protein directly into the bloodstream causes an immune response and symptoms will result.

Leaky Gut Syndrome will present with symptoms such as -

1. Digestive issues including gas, bloating, diarrhoea, constipation or irritable bowel syndrome (IBS).

2. Seasonal allergies or asthma.

3. Hormonal imbalances such as PMS (premenstrual syndrome)or PCOS (polycystic ovary syndrome)

4. Diagnosis of an autoimmune disease such as rheumatoid arthritis, Hashimoto's thyroiditis (where the thyroid destroys itself), lupus, psoriasis, or coeliac disease.

5. Diagnosis of chronic fatigue or fibromyalgia.

6. Mood and mind issues such as depression, anxiety, ADD (attention deficit disorder) or ADHD. (attention deficit hyperactivity disorder)

7. Skin issues such as acne, rosacea, or eczema.

8. Diagnosis of candida overgrowth (see list above)

9. Food allergies and intolerances

The main culprits are foods, infections, and toxins. Gluten is the number one cause of the leaky gut syndrome and this is discussed in depth later in this chapter. Other inflammatory foods such as dairy or toxic foods, like sugar and excessive alcohol, are irritants as well. The most common infectious causes are candida overgrowth, intestinal parasites, and small intestine bacterial overgrowth (SIBO). Toxins come in the form of medications, such as ibuprofen, steroids, antibiotics, and acid-reducing drugs, plus environmental toxins like mercury, pesticides and herbicides especially glyphosate and BPA from plastics. Stress and age also contribute to a leaky gut syndrome.

Healing A leaky Gut

Recovery from this problem is simple but takes effort. First and foremost the pH balance in the bowels needs to be restored, it is important to do everything necessary to prevent creating the acid environment that causes the gut to leak. Simply by changing your dietary choices and sticking to those changes, you will see a profound improvement in a relatively short period of time. Secondly, once you have started improving the pH environment of your bowels, you can help rebuild the "good" bacteria. The best and most effective way to do this is with the aid of a good quality probiotic, preferably one that also contains probiotics - these are non soluble fibre found in very particular foods that provide ideal nutrition for the bacteria in the probiotic. If you are looking for the most effective probiotic you will not find it in the yoghurt-based drinks that can be bought in the supermarket, instead you will be better off taking a Kefir drink, other fermented foods or a supplement. Live bacteria should be stored in the fridge to prolong their effectiveness so if you are buying a supplement off the shelf this may not be the highest quality product. Some exceptions to this exist especially in products that combine pre- and probiotics.

A little word of caution here, it is very easy to create a vicious cycle of poor bowel health if you only use supplementation of probiotics and still keep your diet unhealthy. The bacteria cannot regenerate fast enough between meals to redress the imbalance.

The best approach is to starve the bad bacteria to die off by restricting sugar and yeast and pH-altering foods and support the good bacteria to grow with supplementation.

Probiotics can be taken for life, they are helpful and supportive to your system or they can be used at times of stress to support a tired system.

The more alkaline foods we eat the more likely we are to be healthy on the inside and that will serve us very well. To do this we need to eat many vegetables and fruit each day, we also need to avoid foods that are acidic. Foods sit in categories of acidic, alkaline or neutral. By understanding where a food is on this spectrum you can make smart choices that serve to make you alkaline at every meal. It may take a little time to master the options and understand why you are choosing a particular food but it is well worth the effort.

There are many books written on the acid/alkaline balance and a short internet search will provide charts, recipes and detailed information on just about every food and where it sits on the scale.

There are some fun quirky things to learn with food such as if you test lemon it will register acidic and yet if you drink it infused in water, it alkalises your body!

Allergenic Foods

A true allergy can potentially occur in response to anything, even sunlight, water and air. Some are so severe they are life threatening and must be treated immediately and medically. You may know someone with a true allergy and they carry an epi-pen with them at all times to use if exposed to the trigger allergen.

Allergies show up on the second exposure to the trigger, not the first. The first time a person has exposure, the body mounts a response. This does not show as a serious reaction, usually just a mild reaction or nothing at all however, if that person is exposed a second time, the body is primed immunologically and the response is severe. This second exposure may be the first time someone is even aware there is an issue as that first exposure will have gone pretty well unnoticed.

Food allergies are common; however what is much more common is an intolerance response. People with true allergies have become skilled at avoiding and managing their condition but intolerances can be much harder to identify

An intolerance tends to lead to small and annoying symptoms, a little bit of bloating, indigestion, mild eczema, chronic catarrh, sluggish gut and many many more symptoms.

Most times these warning signs are ignored, yet more often people are tempted to reach for mediation to ease a symptom rather than look for and remove the irritating cause.

Luckily for us many of the foods that are acidic and irritate us through that route are also often the allergenic ones, so simply by eliminating the acidic foods many times you remove allergenic foods as well.

The key culprits (and this in no way is an exclusive list) are dairy, wheat, processed grains, soy, peanuts, eggs and shellfish. An allergic or intolerance response is an immune system reaction. It basically says "I don't like you, you have entered the body and I think you are foreign and no good for me at all, therefore I must destroy you!" It is in that pathway of destruction that all our symptoms occur, either a life-threatening severe reaction with an allergy or a repeating cycle of symptoms associated with an intolerance. In either case, the only way to stop the response is to remove the substance completely.

Elimination diets and then reintegration to monitor responses to certain foods are a fabulous method of identification for intolerances. It is only when the system is "clean" and you then expose it to a food you are intolerant to, that you instantly see the symptom reappear. This way you can see which foods serve you and which foods make you sick.An intolerance is NOT life-threatening, you may eat or drink something that doesn't suit you and the worst that happens is that you feel sluggish, are in pain for a little while, flare up your symptoms or whatever your personal reaction is but it will pass in a relatively short while.

With an allergy you MUST avoid the substance completely and forever, your life can quite literally depend on you doing that.

Addictive Foods

This is a really interesting topic, as there is a distinction between a true addiction and an emotional addiction, they are separate yet intrinsically linked and both driven by the chemical reaction it causes within the body. One is easier to kick than the other and you may be surprised to learn which!

There is also a difference between a craving and an addiction and understanding your own character and what drives your behaviour may help you define where you are on that scale.

The most addictive foods in our modern diets are sugar, coffee, alcohol, carbs (turning into sugar), sweeteners and in addition there are the categories of drugs both prescribed and recreational cause addictions, plus nicotine.

Perhaps surprisingly the emotional addictions are often harder to break than the chemical addictions. Step one requires you to address what is attaching you to that behaviour.

What is your payoff?

Do you find yourself coming in after a stressful day at work and going straight to pour a drink, believing that that relaxes you. Do you munch your way through every evening, does it relieve the boredom? Do you wake and search half asleep for the coffee machine each morning, believing the caffeine is needed to wake you up?

Looking at your behaviours often requires a deep, honest look at yourself and your lifestyle once you have shone some light on your negative behaviour patterns, you will stand half a chance of kicking the attachment to them . It is worth being honest with yourself however painful that may be and discovering why you are driven to a particular food or substance.

Once you get to that point you will find the never ending battle to change suddenly becomes easier. The knowledge alone gives you huge power. It gives you a moment in time to change that behaviour.

Our beliefs drive our thoughts, our thoughts drive our feelings, our feelings drive our behaviours and that loop is what lies behind almost all our conscious actions. The chemical addiction to foods can be changed more simply than you probably realise. In most situations it takes about 48 hours to get the addictive substances chemically out of your system, so physically they are soon gone. Understanding what happens next is key to understanding addiction. Taking sugar as an example is helpful because its use within society is currently at pandemic proportions, it is present in almost every person's diet and it is singularly responsible for more chronic ill health conditions that anything else, so it is worth coming to terms with its addictive nature.

In the simplest form, an addiction is not driven by the substance itself; it is driven by a lack of that substance. It is the change in our body chemistry. Without that substance, it drives us to seek out more to put it back into our bodies. We are looking for relief from the symptoms of lack rather than looking to create the feeling we get with it.

Pleasant as it can be to eat chocolate, the response that drives you to eat more is because the body's reaction to the chocolate wears off, it's the lack of chocolate that makes you want more. If you never had it in the first place you'd never feel the lack, therefore would never want more. It's a vicious cycle once you are exposed to addictive substances.

In the case of sugar – as it is our main source of energy it is a little tricky to avoid. The human body loves to work off glucose, we are programmed for it, we have every system set up for it and when it is in our system, our body can create energy and perform tasks and functions well. If, however, it drops low, we receive signals to seek out more - we may appear hungry, tired and moody.

The relief of those signals comes only from putting more sugar into our bodies and so the cycle begins! The ups and downs, highs and lows of sugar in our bodies drive most people into eating habits that are predictable and unhelpful throughout a day. Someone living off an addition to sugar may have a day that looks something like this -

Mornings will involve carbohydrates for breakfast, either toast, cereals, sweet treats and pastries, tea, coffee, juice.

Mid- morning there will be a slump - biscuits, chocolate even fruit with another stimulant drink will perk you up enough to get you through to lunch

Lunch will consist of sandwiches, wraps, sweet treats, crisps, sweet drinks

Mid afternoon - that slump will drive you to the biscuit tin again and for a few hours until dinner you may be able to stave off that tired feeling

Dinner will often be pasta based or another carbohydrate such as rice, potatoes or bread or a ready meal for convenience and another sugar hit.

Finally, the munchies will set in an hour or two after dinner with a last shot of something sweet before bed.

This is a sugar based diet, with peaks and troughs in your blood sugar levels all day. This is an exhausting and stress-inducing way to live. Each time you are driven to more sugar, it is the need to ease a symptom of your low blood sugar levels that drives your decisions. Any dip will drive a response to find more.

This is how an addition works.

The smoker finds relief from the nicotine levels in their blood dropping by having another cigarette, the drinker by having another drink, the diet soda drinker by having another soda, the coffee drinker by having another coffee.

If you never had these things, if you never developed the reaction in your body on exposure to them it would be impossible for your body to react to the lack of that substance.

If you are a non-smoker you will know exactly what this feels like, You never feel a need for a cigarette because your body has never experienced the chemical response from having one, therefore it cannot drive you to ease the symptom that comes from that lack of a cigarette because it never experienced the chemical change of nicotine in the body in the first place.

Sadly, sugar is everywhere and this is what has made it so deadly to the human body. It is processed, toxic and available to us at an insane level. We should all stand back in absolute amazement that the human body is so miraculous in its adaptive abilities that it can actually survive the assault from sugar for as many years as it does before symptoms show up and the results become life-threatening in the form of diabetes.

These three factors - addictive, allergenic and acidic foods are jointly responsible for a huge part of the chemical stress-load on our bodies. A food diary detailing every food item, drink and drug taken over a week can be an eye-opener for many people, as daily patterns emerge - and from that understanding, real change can begin. It is not uncommon for people to genuinely feel they have a healthy diet until they look back over a food diary with a better understanding of the foods that serve us and the foods that do not. It is at that point that the realisation of some problem areas becomes evident.

In the next few chapters, I am going to explore some key food groups and explain why we ideally need to eliminate them or drastically reduce them in order to regain balance in our bodies and see health return.

CHAPTER 5
Dairy

This is a very emotive topic and yet once the information has been grasped it can hugely benefit health. There is a myth that needs to be blown away, one that has been spread by probably every adult figure in your life, for all of your life. Two facts have been taken, two complete truths and they have been added together and marketed to you so now they are ingrained in your belief system and it is going to take an enormous leap of faith for you to believe anything different. However, stick with the process and you may be surprised by your own shift in belief.

Fact 1 – your bones and teeth need calcium for strength

Fact 2 – dairy products contain calcium

Add these facts together and what do you get?.............. The Dairy industry!

A great starting point for this debate is to ask yourself the question...

"Can you name one mammalian species on this planet that naturally drinks milk past infancy?" i.e. weaning (domesticated cats and dogs do so because we choose what they eat, they don't count!)

The bones and teeth of great apes and elephants would be considered as some of the largest and strongest on earth. Yet, if our bones and teeth crumbled without dairy how do you explain this? How much milk do these animals drink each day to keep them so strong? And their amazingly dense, powerful, strong bones, how does that happen without milk, yoghurt or cheese daily?

The answer is, of course, that their diet does contain the calcium needed for this immense bone strength and interestingly it is not from milk. Their secret food is green leafy vegetation, packed with calcium and other amazing nutrients. It keeps their pH perfect and delivers all the calcium they need in the form they can utilise most effectively.

If you turn your attention now to the milk we primarily choose to drink, you will see there are some major differences between a human being and the species whose milk we choose to drink. Cows have a four-stage stomach, they weigh approximately 90lbs at birth, they gain about 3lbs of weight per day in the first 90 days and weigh about 1,500lbs at 2-3 years old. They are total herbivores, humans are omnivores and even though raw milk is not the worst product for us, pasteurised milk and the processing of raw milk offers many challenges to us on the health front. Until we domesticated animals, our bodies had never even been exposed to cow's milk. We have a blueprint for foods to eat and we are preprogrammed to be able to digest these effectively and utilise their parts for our own growth and regeneration.

Foods that form the perfect diet for us and became part of that blueprint were created about 10,000 years ago, before we domesticated animals for their milk.

There are some very interesting stages in human development; we are first born to a mother who produces milk for us, this happens within the entire spectrum of mammals on this planet. Over time the need for this as a food source changes, teeth erupt and the acid concentration in our stomach rises. These phases are absolutely necessary in preparation for the digestion of other foods. This is the phase and process we call weaning and we understand that this is a transitional phase from a mother totally feeding a baby, to a degree of independence for the child.

Milk contains casein, it also contains calcium. These two substances are linked together chemically and require certain digestive enzymes to break them apart. These enzymes are rennin and lactase. As a human we only have these enzymes for approximately the first three years of our lives, this perfectly covers the period until we are weaned or until we wouldn't be exposed to milk anymore. Upsetting this arrangement is causing the human species many unnecessary health issues.

Dairy is very mucus-forming and as such has been linked to health issues including asthma and a range of digestive conditions. It is often very difficult for us to link the consumption of dairy in our diets to the symptoms it creates as for so many years we have been told to link these products with only good health outcomes, like strong teeth and bones. The dairy industry even managed at one time to convince us to give children a quarter of a pint of milk at school each day. Thankfully this practice was stopped as it was costly and showed no health benefit at all. It did, in my opinion, cause many health issues in an entire generation of children.

Alarming facts about milk..

Not just a glass of goodness! The average glass of milk has been shown to contain an absolute plethora of hormones including pituitary, thyroid, steroid, hypothalamic, parathyroid, growth factors other biologically active substances that are unidentifiable.

Pus cells – UK cows suffer with a variety of infectious diseases, including brucellosis, bovine TB, Foot and Mouth, viral pneumonia and Johne's disease. The cows produce increased white blood cells in response to an infection. These along with cellular debris and dead tissue i.e. somatic cells and pus are excreted into the milk. EU regulations in 1995 set the upper white cell limit at 400,000 cells/mL of milk, primarily as an indicator of the level of bacterial infection present in the mammary glands. This means that up to 4 million pus cells/litre are legally allowable for human consumption!

Antibiotics – sickly cows also mean a constant supply of antibiotics is needed.

Recombinant Bovine Somatotropin (rBST) – in 1994 the Federal Drugs Agency (FDA) in the USA approved the use of this genetically engineered hormone in cows to increase their milk production. Cows given this hormone have elevated levels of insulin-like growth factor, which is linked to certain cancers. Fortunately, the EU, Canada, Japan and more than 100 other countries banned the rBST milk because of its effects on animal health and welfare (not human welfare!!). Worryingly though, the UK still imports dairy products from the US. The expected life span of a dairy cow is cut down drastically from a natural lifespan of 15 years to just 4 years, before they are slaughtered and their meat enters the human food chain.

From cows to children...

Raw milk is collected from farms daily (or every other day) and is transported to dairies by tanker. It is stored at 6°C or less. The milk we drink is heat treated; this includes pasteurisation, sterilisation and UHT (ultra-high temperature) with the aim of making it safe to drink. Many nutrients in milk are destroyed by these heating processes. One important point is that through this process, the milk is being changed from a whole natural food to something that is now altered and unrecognisable to the body. It has limited nutritional value and is no longer viewed as a whole food.

Milk is then separated into different sorts of products, some with fat, some without. Most milk is also homogenised, this is when fat is broken up and dispersed evenly through the product. Milk is finally heated to 72°C then very quickly cooled and stored; this prolongs its shelf life.

The entire process is far removed from how nature intended the milk to be drunk and by whom.

As a footnote, natural, raw untreated milk would be less damaging on the human system than processed milk now is. It would be classed as a non-food rather than a toxic food. Ideally the raw milk would need to be taken from a healthy, grass fed, antibiotic and hormone free-cow, and that is a very rare find in the world today.

IN SUMMARY: COW'S MILK IS MEANT FOR A CALF – NOT A HUMAN

An Interesting Link to Osteoporosis

Human beings are now the only species on earth with osteoporosis (with the exception of cattle and our pets that are now showing with this disease following a prolonged period of being grain-fed; this causes acidity in their bodies). Ironically, the very disease we are trying to prevent is the very disease we are causing. Our fear of weak bones and the message we are told about milk containing the calcium we need to keep our bones strong, appears to fall apart when the facts are examined. We do need calcium to keep our bones and teeth strong; we just need to source it from the correct place, in a form we are programmed to receive it from. We have been so busy worrying where we are going to get our calcium from that we forget to ask the most important question "what is robbing us of the calcium we have?".

Our consumption of calcium through dairy foods has gone up exponentially in the last 30 years. Interestingly, there has been an increased occurrence of osteoporosis in recent decades, too. It is very likely that we have been so busy treating one symptom, that we have completely missed the cause. If we can help people make a smarter choice about their calcium-containing foods and suggest foods that not only provide the body with all the calcium it needs but provide it in an environment that is supportive and healthy and allows the body to utilise the calcium and store it where necessary, then we will be helping the body eliminate toxins and address sufficiency. Dairy is not just in milk, it is in almost all processed foods, chocolate, biscuits, pastries, sauces as well as all the known associated dairy products such as cheese, ice-cream, yoghurt and cream. It is not the worst food on our shelves, it doesn't do as much damage as sugar for example, but as a staple in our daily food intake it is unnecessary and causes a build-up of mucus throughout our bodies and an acidity that makes us sick. Eliminating it for a period of time can very quickly show you how well you can feel without this irritant in your diet. Using plant based milks as an alternative is most helpful and ensuring a daily supply of green leafy vegetables and especially broccoli and spinach and kale will help towards maintaining high and healthy calcium levels.

Processed Grains

Wheat is our most prevalently ingested grain, the most processed and therefore the most damaging to our health.

Just to illustrate what happens to wheat inside the digestive system, take a slice of bread, add a little water, stir it to a pulp just as your stomach would do and then.................... put up some wallpaper! Congratulations, you've just made glue!

Without exaggeration, this is what happens to processed wheat inside you. The human digestive system was never programmed to digest such a material, in fact until the agricultural revolution, these food staples never made it into our diets.

It must be remembered that wheat is a carbohydrate and a refined one at that. It is an insulin-producing, fat-causing, energy-zapping, stomach-bloating, paste-forming, empty drug-like food that keeps people addicted, overweight, and lethargic.

One of the biggest problems with wheat is gas formation, with regular exposure to wheat- based foods the content of our guts literally starts to ferment, have you ever noticed how bloated you are after a bowl of pasta? Yet, this isn't so obvious when you eat rice (2 billion Chinese people can't be wrong!) Another serious concern with wheat is its yeast content.

Over consumption of yeast causes an overgrowth in the microflora of our bowel, creating an imbalance with more "bad" bacteria than good. The more you feed them, the more they grow. If you crave carbohydrates, it is almost certain you are not satisfying your hunger when you eat but are instead feeding the overgrowth of yeast, sugar and wheat- dependent organisms inside your gut.

Imagine a green mould, such as you get on old bread. Now imagine that mould inside your bowel with living organisms buried within it – welcome to Candida. All white refined carbohydrates help to feed these organisms as does milk and sugar. The best approach to getting rid of them is to starve them. Take away the food sources they need to thrive and take a good quality probiotic to replenish the "good" bacteria. I would refrain from reaching for the sweet yoghurt drink probiotics. These are marketed to us from large companies aiming to make profit but it is at the expense of your health.

True Carbohydrates are designed to supply the body with energy, vitamins, minerals, essential fats and amino acids, fibre and water i.e all the building blocks for our growth and wellbeing. Ideally, they are supplied to the body in the form of fruits and vegetables, in this form we get all the nutrients and all the water we need. However, complex manufactured carbohydrates are lacking in water and nutrients. They would be better referred to as just carbs as the hydrate part is completely untrue.

All white refined flour, wheat, pasta, bread, cakes, biscuits and sugar would be best avoided. These foods are toxic, they contribute to weight gain, cause sugar spikes in the blood, chronic ill health and deficiency in essential nutrients. Better alternatives are whole organic oats, wholegrain organic brown rice, rye, spelt, pumpernickel, buckwheat and quinoa. These are best eaten a maximum of once a day in small portions and consumed with water-rich foods such as fruits and vegetables.

The lie that's making you fat...

Carbohydrates are the main source of energy for human beings - and our food choices should reflect that. Below are two representations of our food plate, one based on a standard modern diet and the other an ideal diet.

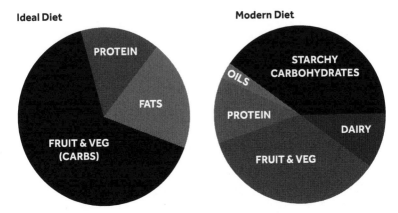

Ideal Diet

PROTEIN

FATS

FRUIT & VEG
(CARBS)

Modern Diet

STARCHY
CARBOHYDRATES

OILS

PROTEIN

DAIRY

FRUIT & VEG

The received wisdom for decades now has been we must cut fat out of our diet because fat makes us fat and unhealthy, choose low fat options and you will decrease your chance of heart disease and stroke, lower cholesterol and prevent weight gain. Well the big news is it is not fat that makes us fat, it is refined carbohydrates. Let me explain...

All excess carbohydrates are stored as glycogen, chemically that is seen as glucose with three fatty acids attached.

Glycogen is stored in the liver and muscle tissue; however storage in these areas is limited to just enough for 24 hours at a time. If we ingest more than we need or can store, the body copes with it by depositing the glycogen in fat cells (adipose tissue). Here's the clever bit, if we have to store a lot of glycogen we just make more fat cells to store it in.

So eating excess carbs makes us store fat.

How do farmers make their cow's fat?..Feed them grains! A little word of caution here: if you are cutting refined carbohydrates out of your diet and yet still eating meat that has been grain-fed, you may be surprised how the negative effect of grain-fed meats can still have an impact on your health. The best option when making a choice on meat is to source grass fed, hormone free, antibiotic-free organic meats. Game meats such as venison, pheasant, even lamb, are much healthier options than beef, chicken or pork.

As a little side note, pork and all pig-based products are best avoided as their flesh is the most similar to human flesh and as such it is very difficult for us to digest. The pectin in apple can help break down the pork, that's why it's always best to eat pork with apple- based condiments or to drink apple juice or even cider with pork.

Choosing different meals, such as soups and salads instead of sandwiches can be easier than compromising on your favourite bread or pasta meal. Eliminating processed grains for four weeks will almost certainly give you improved bowel actions, more energy, less bloating and less abdominal pain as well as almost certain weight loss. Grains have a profound effect on bowel actions primarily because of their glue-like properties and they have a tendency to wreak havoc on the guts. Once you cut back on the constant input of grain, your gut will become much healthier and this will be seen in improved bowel actions. You may not realise what normal bowel activity is, you may just be very used to your own regular pattern and view that as normal. Many people are surprised to learn that normal bowel action is two or more soft,easy to pass bowel actions a day. It is estimated that over 70% of the population suffers with constipation and most people are unaware that their bowel action is sluggish.

Normal bowel activity is only achievable with a balanced, healthy diet. Eliminating processed grains takes you a massive step closer to that.

Gluten

I'm just going to take a moment here to separate wheat from gluten and shine the light purely on gluten. Gluten is so named because of the glue-like properties it possesses. It is a protein composite found in wheat, rye, barley, oats and spelt.

So many foods are now labelled either as gluten-free or containing gluten. This acts as a warning to those with either allergies or intolerances to this irritant. When gluten reaches the digestive tract, it is not unusual for immune cells to mistakenly believe that the protein of gluten is some sort of foreign body, like a bacteria. In certain people who are sensitive to gluten, this causes the immune system to mount an attack against it.

In Coeliac disease (the most severe form of gluten sensitivity), the immune system attacks the gluten proteins, but it also attacks an enzyme in the cells of the digestive tract called transglutaminase. The attack is not only against the gluten protein molecules but also the gut wall itself. This is why Coeliac disease is classed as an autoimmune disorder.

There are many lower-level adverse reactions to gluten and these are termed gluten sensitivity, or gluten intolerance.

Although there is no clear definition of gluten sensitivity, it basically means having some sort of adverse reaction to gluten and an improvement in symptoms on a gluten-free diet.

If you have adverse reactions to gluten, but Coeliac disease is ruled out, then it is called non-coeliac gluten sensitivity.

In non-coeliac gluten sensitivity, there is no attack on the body's own tissues. However, many of the symptoms are similar to those in Coeliac disease, including bloating, stomach pain, fatigue, diarrhoea, as well as pain in the bones and joints.

Unfortunately, because there is no clear way of diagnosing gluten sensitivity, reliable numbers on how common it is are impossible to find. It is estimated that it is affecting more than 40% of the population now.

If you suspect you are sensitive to gluten, eliminate it for 30 days and see how you feel, then reintroduce it again and see how you feel. Symptoms which had disappeared will reappear quickly if you are intolerant to it. The discomfort felt from these digestive upsets can be more than enough to keep you off gluten for life.

Fish

On the plus side, fish creates less acidity in our bodies than red meats. It has zero wheat content, unless it is coated in breadcrumbs or batter, however it is not without issues. Tuna and swordfish should be eaten with caution as they contain a high level of mercury, this is due to the toxicity in our seas and the fact they bioaccumulate toxins as they eat the smaller fish over many years. The recommended consumption would be no more than twice a month to ensure heavy metal exposure stays low enough for our bodies to process. If you love your daily tuna sandwich, you now may be thinking this is something you would be willing to change.

Shellfish is also a poor option as they are bottom feeders and are exposed to many toxins that we then ingest once the fish is eaten. Whilst the protein in fish is exceptionally good for us, sourcing the fish from toxin-free seas is harder than it sounds. Land farmed fish is extremely problematic and the country of origin is relevant when considering the purity of the fish you are buying.

Artificial Sweeteners

These are, as their name suggests artificial - they are man-made. They were accidentally discovered in a laboratory and an idea was born to manufacture them and add them to our food as sweeteners. They offered zero calories and in a world obsessed with calories, zero was a good marketing tool! Manufactured by large companies to improve their profit lines, an extremely toxic carcinogenic substance has made its way into our food chains. In the USA there have been numerous legal actions mounted to try and ban their use. The story behind these battles is quite alarming and a short internet search will provide you with the history. The following summary of facts is intended both as a reference and to shock!!

Artificial sweeteners go by others names such as Aspartame, Splenda, Nutrasweet, Equal, Saccharin, Sorbitol and some very clever e-number disguises, all trying to hide the horrors of the poison being sold to us. In 2008, more than 6,000 common food products were found to contain aspartame. Over 100 countries sell products containing this chemical and more than 250 million people consume it.

So what is aspartame? It consists of three compounds -

Phenylalanine -50% by weigh

Aspartic acid – 40%

Methanol – 10%

Phenylalanine and aspartic acid are amino acids. In aspartame they are joined by a chemical "ester" bond. Once in the body, this chemical bond is broken and the "free forms" cause neurotoxic effects such as headaches, mental confusion, dizziness and even seizures. These chemicals have the alarming ability to cross the blood-brain barrier and cause neuroexcitation of the brain cells. This means the brain cells are over stimulated, over-excited and literally vibrate themselves to death!

The other constituent of aspartame, methanol (wood alcohol) is defined by the FDA (Food and Drug Administration) as having a safe limit of 7.8mg a day, which is about half a can of diet soda. Methanol can spontaneously break down to form formaldehyde, a product found in paint striper and embalming fluid!

The EPA (Environmental Protection Agency) has determined that formaldehyde causes cancer in humans, especially breast and prostate cancer.

They also confirm there is no safe level of formaldehyde in your body. Formaldehyde is stored in the body's fat cells, especially around the hips and thighs. If you keep putting this toxin into your body it has no choice but to keep storing it in fat cells in those areas. You get fatter!

Scientific studies are proving a very strong link between Lupus and MS and diet soda drinkers.

Other common symptoms of aspartame poisoning are leg cramps, vertigo, tinnitus, joint pain, unexplainable depression, anxiety attacks, slurred speech, blurred vision and memory loss.

Aspartame is especially dangerous for diabetics as it disrupts the control of blood sugars and yet is the sugar substitute found in most diabetic foods!

Aspartame passes through the protective blood/brain barrier and damages the neurons in the brain.

This occurs in anyone consuming aspartame but in diabetics the effects are more severe. ADD (Attention Deficit Disorder) and ADHD (Attention Deficit Hyperactivity Disorder) have very strong links to aspartame consumption. In many cases the symptoms completely resolve once the sweeteners are removed from the diet.

Children are at much higher risk and I would suggest they **NEVER** be given artificial sweeteners, yet ironically they are a demographic that are often given them in preference to natural sugars. A decision driven by dental health not brain heath.

A testimonial for life after sweeteners

After a period of time without these toxins you will realise how many day to day symptoms were caused by them. You can read many amazing stories of health recovery that have been reported after withdrawing from aspartame. A story was shared with me many years ago and it is included it here as it highlights the severe effect this chemical can have on our bodies and the amazing recoveries that are possible once it is removed.

"In October of 2001, my sister started getting very sick. She had stomach spasms and she was having a hard time getting around. Walking was a major chore. It took everything she had just to get out of bed; she was in so much pain.

By March 2002, she had undergone several tissue and muscle biopsies and was on 24 various prescription medications. The doctors could not determine what was wrong with her. She was in so much pain, and so sick. She just knew she was dying. She put her house up for sale, sorted her bank accounts, life insurance, etc., and put them in her oldest daughter's name, and made sure that her younger children were to be taken care of.

She also wanted her last hooray, so she planned a trip to Florida (basically in a wheelchair) for March 22nd.

On March 19th I called her to ask how her most recent tests went, and she said they didn't find anything on the test, but they believe she had MS.?

I recalled an article a friend of mine e-mailed to me and I asked my sister if she drank diet soda? She told me that she did. As a matter of fact, she was getting ready to crack one open that moment. I told her not to open it, and to stop drinking the diet soda! I emailed her the article my friend, a lawyer, had sent.

My sister called me within 36 hours after our phone conversation and told me she had stopped drinking the diet soda AND she could walk! The muscle spasms went away. She said she didn't feel 100% but she sure felt a lot better. She told me she was going to her doctor with this article and would call me when she got home.

Well, she called me, and said her doctor was amazed! He is going to call all of his MS patients to find out if they consumed artificial sweeteners of any kind.

In a nutshell, she was being poisoned by the Aspartame in the diet soda...and literally dying a slow and miserable death.

When she got to Florida March 22, all she had to take was one pill, and that was a pill for the Aspartame poisoning! She is well on her way to a complete recovery.

And she is walking! No wheelchair!

If it says 'SUGAR FREE' on the label; DO NOT EVEN THINK ABOUT IT!"

Manufacturers can produce cheap, addictive foods by adding aspartame, it's a win, win situation for them but a complete lose, lose situation for the consumer. Key foods to watch out for are sweets especially coloured fruit ones, chewing gum, anything that says sugar-free on the label, all diet drinks and some non-diet sodas, it is also hidden in many food stuffs especially processed cakes, biscuits and pastries, medicines especially those for children and chewable supplements contain it, plus toothpaste. It is a sound policy to look critically at your food choices and check all labels for sweeteners. If you find them, just throw them out and try to make some different choices next time you are shopping.

If you have a high level in your diet, for example you may be a high level diet soda drinker or chew gum all day, in which case you are likely to feel the effects of withdrawal from the toxins. These usually show as as headaches and thirst, sometimes mood swings and tiredness. The good news is that these withdrawal symptoms are short lived, lasting usually only a few days. Keep your water intake high as it helps flush out toxins and eat as much healthy food as you can manage as you attempt to break the habit and get the toxins out of your system.

Pesticides, Herbicides and GMO

These are a more sinister group of toxins to consider, primarily because they are completely out of our control, crops can be sprayed with chemicals and no mention of their use has to be declared on any packaging of any food substance. Laws are different in different countries and this adds to confusion.

The term GMO will be familiar to most of you and these agents must be considered as they are intrinsically linked to the use of pesticides and herbicides in modern food production.

A genetically modified organism, or GMO, is an organism that has had its DNA altered or modified in some way through genetic engineering. The reason this has become necessary is to improve crop resilience to herbicides and pesticides, thereby increasing the crop yields and farmers' profits. The commonest crops to be affected in this way are high cash crops like soybean, corn, canola and cotton and its obvious to see the appeal from the farming aspect, higher yields, no weeds, pesticide-resistant crops, it all sounds positive, except that those crops are absorbing whatever is being sprayed on them and hence people are consuming the same toxins that are killing everything else they have contact with. Growing a GMO crop basically means it can be sprayed with anything toxic and it will still grow,   only the weeds die.

Commercial sale of GMO foods began in 1994 and it has been controversial since that day. Huge companies sit behind the development of these crops and they have influence at high Government levels and profit is placed well before health. The truth is nobody knows what the long term effects of consuming GMO foods are and forcing transparency on labelling is proving hard. However many health conscious companies choose to label their foods GMO free to let people make their own decisions.

Glyphosate is a herbicide and the main constituent of Roundup, manufactured by Monsanto in the USA. It is also the chemical that is found in Roundup Ready genetically modified seeds. Think of it as creating a seed that is already impregnated with the chemical toxin to kill any pest or weed that would even think about attacking the developing plant. It is "born" ready to resist the toxin by containing the toxin in the first place.

Americans have applied 1.8 million tons of glyphosate since its introduction in 1974.

Worldwide 9.4 million tons of the chemical has been sprayed on fields –

enough to spray nearly half a pound of Roundup on every cultivated acre of land in the world.

Globally, glyphosate use has risen almost 15-fold since so-called "Roundup

Ready,"genetically engineered glyphosate-tolerant crops" were introduced in 1996.

In 2015, the World Health Organisation declared Glyphosate "probably a strong carcinogen" meaning it can cause cancer.

On March 28, 2017, the California Environmental Protection Agency's Office of Environmental Health Hazard Assessment confirmed that it would add glyphosate to California's Proposition 65 list of chemicals known to cause cancer. Monsanto sued to block the action but the case was just dismissed. Money can buy silence and a lot of money is thrown at quieting all rumours that threaten the profit lines from the sale of both the seeds and the spray.

The battle goes on between people suing Monsanto, Government legislation, scientific research, lobbies, cover ups and corruption and somewhere in amongst all the debate, there is the truth. I would strongly advise you to research this chemical and make up your own mind and then make your own choice on the foods that you buy, companies that you support and research that you believe.

My decision will be to always eat GMO free, to fight for transparent labelling and to be very dubious about any company that has enough money and power to manipulate Governments and scientific data.

Soya

From the early 1990's there was a directed campaign by the Soya industry to put their products at the forefront of healthy decision making. It was strongly marketed as a healthy food option and the benefits of phytoestrogens touted across the media. This led to a huge surge in sales and made soya a popular and common place product.

Unfortunately, the evidence does not support the claims and soya has a severe hidden sting. It affects hormones. Being high in plant-based oestrogen, it disrupts the hormone balance in the body and it is particularly bad for men. First suggested as a beneficial food for menopausal women, with the supposed health benefit of consuming plant-based oestrogen, it was a logical and simple beneficial idea to buy in to.

Common health issues related to soya products are malnutrition, digestive distress, immune-system breakdown, thyroid dysfunction, cognitive decline, reproductive disorders and infertility - even cancer and heart disease.

The vast majority of soya available at health food shops or the supermarket is not to be viewed as a health food. The exception is fermented soya, which is discussed below.

To make a problem food even worse, there is now GMO soya that is contaminated with large pesticide and herbicide residues. The reason they have made it GMO, is so they can spray the potent toxic herbicide Roundup (Glyphosate) on them to improve crop production by killing the weeds.

In the Asian culture, people eat small amounts of whole non-GMO soybean products as well as fermented soy products such as soy-sauce, tempeh, miso and natto - all with health benefits and none of the toxic effects of processed soya found in the western world. Another issue in the west is the separation of the soybean into two commodities -protein and oil - there is nothing natural or safe about these products.

The perception of these products as healthy is a major issue and what is needed above all else is education on soya, fermented soya, GMO soya and what our health choices actually should include. Please become a label reader for soya products and derivatives and avoid them as much as possible.

Finally on this topic, it is important to consider animal feed, even if you are not personally choosing to eat soya-based products, they are being fed to animals as feed so unless you source meat that has come from grass-fed animals, you may still be ingesting a high level of GMO soya via the meat you are eating. Eighty percent of the world soya crop goes to animal feed!

To conclude on soya

- More than 90% of US-grown soya is from GM crops

- Soya contains a natural toxin called an anti-nutrient, these interfere with enzymes used to digest proteins

- Soya contains phytates, these prevent certain minerals from being absorbed

- Soya contains goitrogens which block the function of the thyroid gland

- Soya contains hemagglutinin causing red blood cells to clump together

- Soya contains isoflavones, a type of phytoestrogen which is very disruptive to hormone function

- Soya contains high levels of aluminium and manganese

- Soya infant formula is to be avoided it has been shown to irreversibly damage the reproductive system of developing infants.

There are so many wonderful alternatives available now, with plant and nut-based milks available on our supermarket shelves. There is a strong move towards vegan and vegetarian diets which help to cut down the exposure to these foods via meat. Many foods become popular due to marketing and publicity driven by the companies producing those products. Basically, they just want to persuade you to buy their products. Yet remember you retain a phenomenal power to place your purchasing power where YOU choose. If enough people make a shift, change will happen!

CHAPTER 6

Diabetes

Diabetes is a disorder of sugar metabolism which exists in two forms – type 1 and type 2. Type 1 is an autoimmune disorder and represents a failure of the pancreas to produce insulin. As insulin is the hormone that lowers blood sugar levels, the body's inability to produce it in type 1 diabetes leads to a critical situation that if left untreated, is life- threatening. The solution with type 1 diabetes is to provide the body with carefully controlled, self-administered amounts of insulin, delivered by injection or pump driver. Sugar intake is critical and people with type 1 diabetes become experts at controlling and monitoring their condition.

Type 2 diabetes is a completely different disorder. It is chronic in onset and caused entirely by many years, often decades, of dietary self-abuse and poor lifestyle choices. By definition it is therefore preventable by avoiding those underlying causal factors.

Type 2 diabetes used to be termed mature onset diabetes, giving a clue as to the demographic that develops the disorder. It is a sad state of affairs that due to the ever lower age group that is being diagnosed with this type of diabetes, the name has now been changed. It is quite alarming how many children are now diagnosed with it and there is evidence that babies are born with type 2 diabetes if their mother's diet has been poor enough for long enough.

Who gets it?

The single greatest indicator of risk is weight. Others factors include age (being over 40 immediately places you in a higher risk category) and ethnic background also has an influence.

Statistics

Due to the close relationship between obesity and diabetes, there are two statistics that should be considered, firstly the incidence of obesity within a society and secondly the incidence of the actual disease, diabetes.

1 in 10 people in the UK are clinically obese.

1 in 4 people have weight issues, placing the UK in second position for obesity on the world stage.

In the 1980's, six per cent of men and eight per cent of women were classed as obese. In 2017, 24% men and 26% women were in that category - tripling the incidence in just over 30 years!

In children across both genders, the incidence is now 3 in 10 for obesity.

Following current rates, it is predicted that by 2030, 11 million people in the UK will be obese.

The UK currently spends 48 billion pounds per year on health and social services related entirely to weight issues in the population.

This rising obesity epidemic is predicted to be responsible for an additional 7 million cases of diabetes, 6.5 million cases of stroke and heart disease and half a million cases of cancer by 2030.

It is predicted that by 2050, one in three adults will have diabetes caused entirely by weight issues.

These statistics are from the World Health Organisation, Diabetes UK and the CDC (Centre for Disease Control and Prevention) and are readily available to view online each year. They are comparable to other westernised countries and run almost parallel to US statistics for these disorders. Obesity and diabetes are causing extreme concern within health circles as their prevalence is now so high that treating the disorders themselves and the complications from them is, within a few years, going to prove the downfall of many health services worldwide.

Addressing the causes as early as possible and preventing the onset is the only sensible approach. However, getting people to engage in different behaviours is proving much more difficult than originally expected. A lifetime of bad eating and lifestyle habits, as well as the availability of processed foods, combine to produce a dreaded disease but people are still reluctant to admit that their day-to-day food and exercise choices are having such a serious impact on their health.

Obesity alone brings many challenges each day and people suffer with social stigma as well as mental and physical stress as a result of weight issues. Knowing you have weight issues does not in itself help you deal with them. Education will play an incredibly important role in changing society's perception of health and how to achieve it. The primary approach for obesity and diabetes is dietary and lifestyle changes. It makes more sense to address these as good lifestyle choices and prevent the onset of these conditions in the first place. If you're going to have to address your weight, food and exercise routines when you are diagnosed with the problems anyway, you might as well do it now and prevent the disease. That would be my view.

Obesity and Diabetes

The link between diabetes and obesity is not even questionable, such is the strength of the evidence. What is a little more uncertain, is exactly how the physiology of the body is behaving to create such a strong connection. One theory that is being addressed currently and researched quite heavily is the involvement of a hormone called leptin. Early results from these studies are showing that it may be the missing link between why weight issues turn into diabetes.

Without any doubt insulin is the key player. As blood sugar levels rise, insulin is released to bring them back down. However, science has always struggled to complete all the pieces in this puzzle and so the diabetes and obesity epidemic has never been completely understood.

What Role Might Leptin Play?

Leptin is a protein hormone that plays a key role in regulating energy intake and energy expenditure, including appetite and metabolism. Leptin was discovered in 1994 by Jeffrey M. Friedman and colleagues at the Rockefeller University through the study of obese mice.

Human leptin is a protein made up of 167 amino acids. It is manufactured primarily in the fat cells of white adipose tissue, and the level of circulating leptin is directly proportional to the total amount of fat in the body.

Leptin acts on receptors in the hypothalamus of the brain where it inhibits appetite.

The absence of leptin (or its receptor) leads to uncontrolled food intake and resulting obesity.

To date, only leptin and insulin are known to act as a signal to the body to deposit fat.

Leptin is a circulating signal that reduces appetite, but obese individuals generally exhibit an unusually high circulating concentration of leptin. These people are said to be resistant to the effects of leptin, in much the same way that people with type 2 diabetes are resistant to the effects of insulin. The high sustained concentration of leptin from the enlarged fat stores, result in leptin desensitisation. The body keeps pumping out leptin but the body does not "hear" the signal and the result is a situation where there is high fat levels and high leptin levels.

Leptin resistance is sometimes described as a metabolic disorder that contributes to obesity, similar to the way insulin resistance is sometimes described as a metabolic disorder that has the potential to progress into type 2 diabetes. This point is still being researched but it is clear that the metabolic functions of the body become severely compromised in obese individuals and disease will result if the situation is not reversed. Mammalian physiology is always about survival and the current understanding is that our bodies will always act to prolong our survival even at the cost of making us fat or unwell. We are back to our iceberg analogy, where the important change really is getting off the iceberg!

Medicine has not heard the last of leptin, as research continues into it and the exact role it plays in the modern day epidemic of obesity becomes clearer, is it a cause or a result? One thing is certain, as the research narrows down its role, the drug companies will be falling over themselves to create a leptin-based drug with the claim it will solve weight issues. Apply caution and be very wary of this, remember all drugs come with side effects and the only real answer to weight issues is to change what and how you eat, how much exercise you undertake and how you manage your stress levels There really are no short cuts.

Complications of Diabetes

Diabetes comes with a plethora of complications that in many ways are worse than the disease itself. The strain it places on the body leads to system failures and almost certainly premature death.

Possible complications include extreme tiredness, a five-fold increase in cardiovascular disease, retinopathy leading to blindness, sensory, motor or autonomic neuropathy giving the possibility of affecting any nerve conduction anywhere in the body and symptoms such as an inability to perceive hot, cold, pain and touch. The debilitating condition of Charcot's foot commonly presents due to weakness and deformity of the feet. Gastroparesis occurs as the gut becomes sluggish; nausea is common as is bloating, vomiting, diarrhoea, constipation, abdominal pain and unintentional weight loss. Bladder issues show with repeated infections and incontinence as well as erectile dysfunction, impotence, low blood pressure, excess sweating and skin disorders. Severe vascular issues can result and in extreme cases these can lead to gangrene and amputation of limbs.

Why does this all happen?

To understand this it is necessary to know a little about how sugar and insulin are needed and used by the body.

Sugar

Human beings rely very heavily on sugars for energy. Sugars in the form of simple and complex carbohydrates are the most easily used form of energy. Through a series of chemical conversions the body can also utilise fats and proteins but by choice it would use sugar in the form of glucose as its primary energy source. A surplus of glucose in the bloodstream that is not needed for energy will be converted into glycogen and stored in the muscles and liver for future use. Enough energy for 24 hours can be stored this way and the remainder of any excess calories from a carbohydrate diet is converted to fat and stored in the body for future use.

Excess sugars result in fat cells being made to store the excess in.

Insulin

Insulin is a hormone secreted from the pancreas in response to elevated blood sugar levels. As with every function of the body, balance is key and when the body detects elevating blood sugar levels, it responds to lower them again. The higher blood glucose levels rise, the more insulin is produced . This leads to a state where the body has high glucose levels in the blood **and** high insulin levels – this is called **insulin resistance** and is one stage before complete fatigue of the pancreas and the diagnosis of type 2 diabetes.

Both type 1 and type 2 diabetes refer to an inability of the pancreas to produce insulin. What differs is the route to that scenario. One is caused by a predisposition, the other by self destruction.

Within the body insulin has many other uses

It promotes the storage of fat;

It controls the total quantity of protein in the body;

It is used in cell replication;

The immune system needs it

Hormone balance, especially thyroid hormones rely on it

Insulin resistance and type 2 Diabetes lead to –

Pronounced stress response within the body – increased cortisol and adrenalin levels;

Vitamin C deficiency;

Magnesium deficiency;

Increased sodium levels

The scenario of high insulin levels and high glucose levels, leading to insulin resistance, with associated low magnesium and high sodium levels, constricts blood vessels, leads to fluid retention and triggers the stress response; this acts as a perfect precursor to cardiovascular disease.

Defined as Metabolic Disease or Syndrome X, it is the disease of our time. It is caused purely by high sugar diets arising primarily from all the carbohydrates we ingest. Generally we now ingest much more energy than we require on a daily basis and the scenario of weight gain, pancreatic exhaustion, diabetes and the health complications that result can lead to premature death from a disease that is completely preventable by different lifestyle choices.

How to prevent Diabetes

1. Watch your weight
2. Keep your waist measurement below 32inches (81.25cms) for a female and 38inches (96.5cms) for a male
3. Eat fresh fruit and vegetables daily
4. Eat complex carbohydrates
5. Avoid processed sugars, corn syrup and sweeteners
6. Take Omega 3 supplements daily
7. Exercise regularly

Glycaemic index

Glycaemic index, or GI is a measure of the effects of carbohydrates on blood sugar levels. Carbohydrates that break down quickly during digestion and release glucose rapidly into the bloodstream have a high Glycaemic Index; carbohydrates that break down more slowly, releasing glucose more gradually into the bloodstream, have a low Glycaemic Index.

Classification	GI Level	Examples
Low GI	55 or less	most fruits and vegetables, legumes / pulses, whole grains, nuts, fructose and products low in carbohydrates
Medium GI	56 - 69	whole wheat products, basmati rice, sweet potato, sucrose
High GI	70 and above	baked potatoes, watermelon, white bread, most white rices, corn flakes, extruded breakfast cereals, glucose, maltose

The aim should be to eat foods that have a GI of less than 50 and learn to avoid any foods that have a GI above 100.

Diabetics should be wary of consuming too many sugars via fruit. Juices and smoothies represent an amazing source of concentrated live nutrients but they also deliver a high punch of sugars that can elevate blood glucose levels and place an extra strain on an already stressed system. If you are concerned about your sugar intake, buffer your juices with sea algae such as super green foods, spirulina, wheatgrass and omega 3 oil, avocado, soluble fibre, ground linseeds and psyllium husks. Learn to enjoy vegetable- based juices rather than sweet, sugar filled smoothies.

Diabetic foods do not offer a good alternative. They will not improve your blood sugar levels any more than a carefully controlled diet will. They are costly and are often sweetened with artificial sweeteners, which in themselves pose a real threat to your health. (See the earlier chapter for more information on sweeteners and the damage they do to health).

Juice Ideas

DIVINE VEGGIE JUICE

½ large pineapple

2 apples

Handful of alfalfa, watercress, parsley, kale and broccoli

1oz shot of wheatgrass or 1 teaspoon of powdered form

Pack all the veg between 2 apples before you juice.

Place in a blender with ice/water and wheatgrass powder

AVOCADO CREAM WITH LIME

1 avocado

4 apples

½ pineapple

½ cucumber

1 lime (peeled)

Supergreen powder food

Juice the pineapple, apples, cucumber and lime.

Place the avocado and powder in a blender with a little water/ice.

Add the juice to the blender mix and whizz for 30 seconds.

Exercise

This is an incredibly important component in the prevention and treatment of type 2 diabetes and obesity. On a simple equation of calories used against calories eaten, someone who exercises regularly will always use more of their excess energy up and therefore not need to store it.

The type of exercise that works best is interval training where the heart rate rises for a short period of time followed by a rest period, repeated over 30 minutes and done 3-5 times a week. This has been shown by scientific research to lower the chance of developing diabetes and obesity and is a beneficial approach to treating diabetes also.

A brisk 30 minute walk daily lowers the chance of developing diabetes by 91%

The Medical approach to Diabetes treatment

Since the seventies, doctors have recommended a low fat diet for diabetics. They have been aware of the dietary and lifestyle link to the disorder and usually work hard to encourage patients to lose weight and exercise more. The low fat diet was the diet of choice because of the concern doctors had about the increase risk of heart disease. Under the mistaken belief that low-fat diets improve heart disorders, they strongly pushed this as their treatment of choice – how wrong they were!

The other approach, since the introduction of statin drugs, has been to prescribe them for their diabetic patients. This compounds the problem and combined with the low-fat diet advice has caused diabetic patients to deteriorate and often die earlier, from what is an almost 100% preventable and treatable disease with the correct advice.

Early in 2018, Diabetes UK gave its official backing of new advice that a low-fat diet is incorrect, statins are unnecessary and the approach of choice is a low carb diet. Even back as far as 2004, research was clearly showing the amazing benefits to eating a low- carb diet, results as good as a 20% drop in blood sugar levels were seen even after only a few weeks on such a programme. The low-fat diet approach never achieved results that impressive in all the decades it was promoted.

Current thinking and research points ever more towards a plant-based diet and periods of fasting to reverse even severe Type 2 diabetes. No one can claim this is an easy route, it requires willpower and discipline, however the success rates are incredible.

The sad irony to this situation is that if the whole cholesterol paradigm had not been allowed to rule medical belief on heart disease for the last 60 years, it would not have been so wrong with the advice given to diabetics. To understand more about the issues around cholesterol read on as the next chapter will dig deep into fats, statins and the great cholesterol con!

In 2008, The American Diabetic Association changed its advice on low-carb diets and where this advice has been acted on it has shown effective results in weight loss and diabetes control. Sadly, getting doctors to act on this new information has not been so effective. Their reluctance to move away from the high-fat diet causes patients to be fat myth, means the truth around diabetes is proving very difficult to pass on to patients. It is worth investigating the current research, it is moving in the right direction, people are hearing information independently and acting on it with great results and saving their own lives.

If sufferers with Type 2 diabetes, or indeed anybody interested, wants to learn about all the current research, a docu-series by Jon Mahon called 'iThrive' is available online or to own.

There are about nine hours of footage to watch, all of it fully researched and proving time and time again than once you understand the beast that is diabetes, you can beat it!

Low carb does not mean NO carb. Carbohydrates offer a wonderful source of energy and in their natural state still represent the perfect energy source.

Eliminating them completely will cause major health issues – remember Atkins?! Be careful and cautious and do not go for overkill. Sugar issues and therefore weight and diabetic health issues have been caused by dietary abuse for years, very often decades, relying too heavily on processed sugary carbs that cause blood sugar levels to peak and trough. Over years, this fatigues the body to the point of breakdown and illness. Correction is a gradual process of dietary education. Fasting or extremely low-calorie intake diets, often based around vegan protein sources, are proving hugely successful in reversing Type 2 Diabetes in relatively short periods of time.

The dietary advice, following this new directive, is to cut out sugary drinks including fruit juice. Take healthy essential fatty oils such as omega 3, eat lean meats, preferably grass- fed, hormone-free varieties, or better still go completely plant based. Over time, this information will filter through to the GPs and finally there will be a uniform approach to beating such a devastating, but preventable disease.

Other sources of material on diabetes

NICE (National Institute for Clinical Excellence) are releasing new guidelines on the treatment and prevention of diabetes. This information was presented to GPs in 2011. It is hoped that some of the new directives that are now being supported will result in action across the board and that some of the older policies are abandoned immediately.

The emphasis in this report is almost completely on the fact that results will be achieved on prevention of the disease through lifestyle change and also that the treatment of the disease is through lifestyle change. This indicates categorically that this is a disease of modern living and it can be eradicated with changes in lifestyle and improvements in dietary choices and exercise patterns. It seems, finally, there may be some positive-thinking about the advice.

Diabetes UK is the national centre for guidelines and information relating to this disease, its website is user friendly and informative. They offer these new directives their complete support and are working towards new dietary information and more research into the effectiveness of this approach. It will be very hard then for the medical profession not to support it.

Remember...

Diabetes is preventable by lifestyle changes

CHAPTER 7
Cholesterol The Shocking Truth

Cholesterol - the word alone makes you feel you should run to your GP to get your levels checked. Plenty of us do just that and far too many of those patients who go through the GP's door for a check up find themselves coming out with a prescription for statins.

Aside from the fact that the Quality Outcome Framework system financially rewards GPs and their practices for signing people up for statin medication, there is a massive amount of misunderstanding surrounding this fundamental health issue. What if there is even a chance this information could be wrong?

Enormous confusion has developed around the subject of fats, cholesterol, statins, diets and lifestyles and the information as well as being confusing, is even contradictory. Much of this conflicting advice has resulted from a desire by many health practitioners to keep a doubtful hypothesis alive with much "clutching at straws" and development of ad-hoc theories that has diverted attention away from the fact that the cholesterol theory is, in fact, flawed.

It is the ultimate case of square peg and round hole and yet there are a number of institutions that just keep bashing that square peg into that round hole, particularly the drug companies who stand to benefit from the prescriptions being handed out at the GP's surgery.

Dr Malcolm Kendrick in his book 'The Great Cholesterol Con' explores in detail every aspect of the cholesterol myth. For anyone facing decisions about their health in this arena, I highly recommend reading the book before you make any decisions. Knowledge is power, understanding is power.

For a theory to be true and become a known fact, all research, understanding and outcomes must always continue to prove that theory true. ALL facts must fit or else the theory is no longer valid. The cholesterol theory has always been flawed and yet because of the power of lobbies, drug companies and outdated science; powerful and influential people refuse to see all the issues with their line of thinking. What follows below is my attempt to show you the issues with the cholesterol theory and then you can make up your own mind.

The next few pages are rather science-orientated but to truly be able to make the correct health decisions, it is important to understand how and why things happen within the body.

How have we got to this point?

It all began in the mid-19th century when a pathologist, Rudolf Von Virchow, looked down a microscope and saw arteries with plaques containing cholesterol (amazing that he knew how cholesterol looked, but back to the story...). He concluded that the cholesterol he saw must have come from the blood. Despite this discovery, it was 50 years before another step forward (or possibly backwards) was made.

A Russian researcher called Nikolai Anitschkov fed high-cholesterol diets to rabbits and noted that their arteries thickened with plaques filled with cholesterol - he was convinced he had proved that cholesterol in the diet is deadly and causes heart disease.

Or maybe he just proved that rabbits didn't survive well on a carnivore's diet???

Many years passed as people were not that interested in heart disease and edicine was very busy discovering things like germs and how to reduce the mortality rate during surgery.

However, after WWII there seemed to be an increase in deaths from heart disease so interest began to stir, an interest that turned to real concern by the early 1950's when the USA felt it was on the brink of a heart disease epidemic. In a panicked attempt to get some quick answers, they backed a scientific study. This was to become the most quoted study into the cause of heart disease. Published in 1953 by Ancel Keys, it showed the results of a comparison of diets and incidence of heart disease in 22 countries. However, in his report Keys submitted results from only six or seven (this number varies depending on which research you read) of the countries that he studied. He only included those that helped prove his point that high-fat diets cause heart disease, not the other 15 or 16 that showed no correlation at all between dietary fat intake and heart disease. Those were excluded from his results.

These studies were looking at fat intake and its effect on heart disease, not cholesterol and heart disease. The results of this study were pounced upon by the US government as proof of a dietary link to heart disease and the government believed it could at least answer one question now -

"What causes heart disease?"

Without hesitation, the US administration moved forward with its "new theory" that dietary intake of fat clogs arteries and causes heart disease. All that remained to be answered was how to treat it. Enter low-fat foods - something never before seen but worth billions of dollars to the food industry. Then the drug companies developed medication that could treat the disease - another money-spinner.

The results of this study have echoed through decades, never supported by further proof of a causal connection between diet and heart disease and yet disproved dozens of times by well-conducted scientific experiments and culture-based studies from around the world.

To truly understand the details of how such a con can develop read deeper into the subject in the book 'The Great Cholesterol Con', it is an amazing resource, written for medical professionals and the public. In it, he highlights the mistakes made. The book explains why these few countries did, in fact, have an increased rate of heart disease and yet this information is well hidden from public view. In summary, these countries all had large populations, sometimes into the millions, that had been relocated post-war, often to completely different countries - a phenomenon called social dislocation. It is now believed to be the single biggest risk factor for heart disease.

Ignore for a moment all the obvious mistakes that have occurred to scientifically arrive at the conclusion that fat causes heart disease. There still remains a huge question to be answered if Ancel Keys was correct and the fats in our diets are to blame - "How exactly does fat in our diets increase our chance of a heart attack?" I am going to apply a little basic biochemistry as I hope it will help you understand this, although the systems are extremely complex the basic facts are enough to help you understand the principles and that in turn will help you understand the role fats play within the body.

The Different Types of Fats

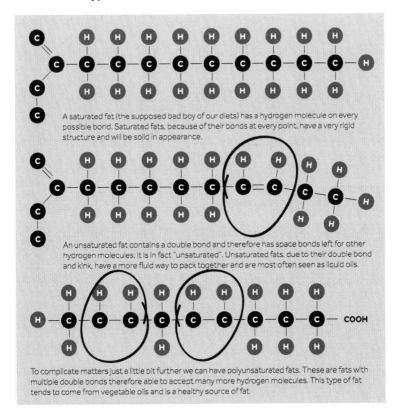

A saturated fat (the supposed bad boy of our diets) has a hydrogen molecule on every possible bond. Saturated fats, because of their bonds at every point, have a very rigid structure and will be solid in appearance.

An unsaturated fat contains a double bond and therefore has space bonds left for other hydrogen molecules; it is in fact "unsaturated". Unsaturated fats, due to their double bond and kink, have a more fluid way to pack together and are most often seen as liquid oils.

To complicate matters just a little bit further we can have polyunsaturated fats. These are fats with multiple double bonds therefore able to accept many more hydrogen molecules. This type of fat tends to come from vegetable oils and is a healthy source of fat.

Unfortunately at this point man intervened, thinking it was a smart idea to try and add hydrogen molecules onto the free bonds of unsaturated fats, so in a process called hydrogenation, hydrogen was fired at the liquid oil of healthy fats at high speed and very high temperatures in the hope that some may became attached! What was found when this was done was that the nice healthy liquid oil with free bonds attached to the hydrogen became solid. Man had created margarine.

Margarine might be easier to spread on toast but it is incredibly unhealthy. When the body encounters substances it doesn't recognise it tends to panic a little, viewing them as unnatural, toxic and dangerous. The body goes into an adaptive state while it tries to deal with the toxic effect and this has health consequences.

In nature, whether the fat is saturated or unsaturated, the hydrogen atoms appear on the same side of the double bond, known as the cis configuration.

Cis Configuration

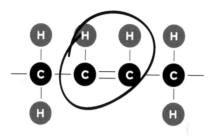

When the hydrogen atoms appear on opposite sides of the double bond, this is known as the trans configuration, and fatty acids containing this configuration are known as trans fatty acids.

Trans Configuration

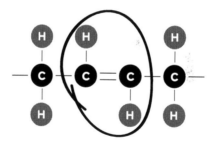

Trans fats

These fats are found in man-made processed foods, not in nature. These are very unhealthy and pressure is growing from health groups and the scientific community to ban them. Trans fats have now been removed from a lot of products and the lobby against them has been strong enough to ban them in some countries. However, they still appear in many familiar products and cause health issues in anyone who eats them, including links to cancer, heart disease, liver disease, diabetes, obesity and fertility issues.

Moving fats around

Fats are insoluble in water and therefore cannot dissolve in the blood, yet they need to be transported around the body. The body solves this problem by forming a triglyceride; this represents '3 fatty acids' (another name for a fat molecule) connected together by a backbone of glycerol (part glucose).

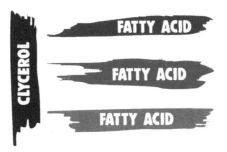

Once they have formed a triglyceride they join with something called a lipoprotein and travel around the body in that way. There are several sizes of lipoprotein, the largest of which is called a chylomicron; the next size down is called a very low density lipoprotein (VLDL); smaller still is an intermediate density lipoprotein (IDL); further down are the two people are most familiar with, low density lipoprotein (LDL the bad boy of the fat world) and high density lipoprotein (HDL-hailed a hero in the fat world!)

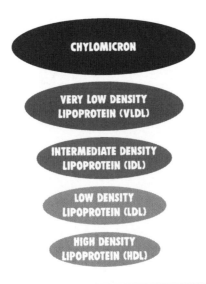

That is about it as far as the story about fats goes.

Still no mention of cholesterol in this science lesson, why? Well, cholesterol really has nothing to do with fat except that it uses the same lipoprotein transport system and travels round the body in the same way. Most lipoprotein picks up fat from around the body, especially the digestive system, muscles and the liver, drops it off where needed and returns to the liver for a reprocessing action. The body is a carefully balanced machine that knows exactly what it is doing. Left unhindered, it will perform to perfection.

So how have we come to believe there is such a strong link between dietary fat and heart disease?

The answer is – we are just being told it by people we have been taught to trust, therefore it becomes believable. When a doctor sits you down and tells you your cholesterol levels are high, all the information you have ever heard supporting this as a dreadful finding will flood into your head and you will look to the doctor for a solution. What you will get is advice on a low-fat diet and a prescription for statin drugs. You have no further information to hand that would make you believe this was not the solution.

However, if you were in possession of real knowledge and understanding of a different reality you may feel very empowered to question their advice.

Bear in mind that GPs get financial payouts for prescribing statin drugs. Due to the one- sided media coverage and the perpetuation of the myth about fat in our diets leading to heart disease they have to do very little except give you a result of a high cholesterol reading to have you fearful of your impending heart attack.

Pausing for a moment to understand more about what is going on in the body and why your cholesterol may be elevated will probably save your life. If, for example, your reading is 7, this may not necessarily be bad news. Your reading could always have been 7 but if this is your first cholesterol test you may not know that. Only an elevation above 7 (or below) would indicate a change and the next most sensible question to ask is "why has that changed?" not "how do we change it"! The number one rule should be to find the cause and not to just treat the symptom. Remember. it's prudent to identify the iceberg before you treat exposure to cold.

WHY Cholesterol is ESSENTIAL to LIFE

What is Cholesterol?

Cholesterol is made from Acetyl CoA which as well as other chemicals, contains phosphorus, sulphur and nitrogen, none of which are found in fats (fats contain carbon, oxygen and hydrogen) Acetyl CoA also has several ring structures rather than the straight molecular structure that is found in all fats. In a very complicated 14-step process, the body takes Acetyl CoA and converts it into cholesterol in the liver. We can ingest some cholesterol in our diets. Our best sources of this are eggs, oils and nuts, but almost invariably people never eat enough each day to fulfil the demand our bodies have for cholesterol, so our bodies make up the difference, not having enough is not an option as so many vital life functions rely on it being present. Here are examples of some of the key functions cholesterol are used for in our bodies -

Brain synapses (connections) – found between cells in the brain, these synapses are almost completely made of cholesterol

Vitamin D – needed to create healthy bones and protect against cancers, it's made from cholesterol after exposure to sunlight.

Cell membranes – 75 trillion cells in your body and they all need cholesterol in their cell membranes.

Sex hormones – all steroid-based hormones require cholesterol in their production

Bile - cholesterol is a key component in bile. Bile is essential in fat metabolism.

What would happen to your brain, body cells, bones, digestion and hormone production if you had no cholesterol? One condition does exist where the body fails to produce cholesterol, called the Smith-Lemli-Opitz Syndrome (SLOS), a disorder that is almost always fatal, proving we need cholesterol. Without it we die!

How can things have got so mixed up and how can we all be jumping on the 'eat bad fat, make cholesterol, clog arteries and die of heart disease' bandwagon?

After years spent researching the topic and working in health and wellness, it is baffling trying to understand the mentality of backing such an obviously flawed hypothesis. The holes in this theory are everywhere, the poor results of treating patients with this approach almost prove the theory is wrong, and yet the "experts" still insist that the theory is correct. If you have any worries about heart disease, education and research will arm you with valuable information.

Why does cholesterol get stuck in our arteries?

This is a really good question. Why does something as helpful and necessary as cholesterol find itself getting stuck in our blood vessels and causing health issues? Hopefully you are starting to consider (if not completely believing yet) the truth that there really is no connection between ingesting healthy fats and heart disease. There are however SERIOUS health consequences to ingesting chemically altered fats. Through exceptionally clever marketing, most people still think choosing low-fat options and margarine over butter is the healthy sensible choice – WRONG! This has been the greatest mistake.

The statistical figures for the incidence of heart disease over the last 30-40 years show it has risen every year. Surely if the right thing were being done by cutting out fat and changing the choices made in the fats being eaten, there would be a year-on-year decrease in the incidence of heart disease? The wrong theory is inevitably producing the wrong result. Some basic facts cannot be disputed. For more than 100 years, cholesterol has been identified in plaques in arteries. The question that should be asked is why does cholesterol appear to get stuck and clog these arteries?

The answer is interesting - the reason we develop plaques and cause blockages is due to the body's stress response and normal physiology being forced to adapt to a stressor. This leads back (as does all chronic illness) to the basics of health.

It is suggested that a lack of vitamin C is at the root of heart disease combined with the fact that we are under continual stress in the modern world (far different from our ancestors' stress).

The system works like this......

There is a cut or tear to the inside of an artery (remember it's a very high pressure system, naturally prone to small areas of damage on a continual basis). Just as a cut on the skin would bleed for a while and then be plugged, the same reaction happens internally. The healing continues under the plug until the artery wall is healed up. Now things get a little different because if that plug/scab fell off as it does on external wounds, it would drift in the blood vessels until it got stuck in a small blood vessel, cause a blockage and a stroke would be the result. So the body has a system. (Yes, it knows what to do without a drug telling it how to behave! It's a miracle!) Millions of progenitor cells (from the bone marrow) circulate in the bloodstream and when there is a breach in an artery wall they try and cover it up. However, the clot (containing cholesterol) has often got there first and these cells form on top of the clot, they create a new cell wall and the clot is forced backwards into the wall of the blood vessels and not pushed off into the bloodstream. A very, very clever system.

The reason cholesterol is linked into this system at all is the fact that cholesterol is used in the healing process. It is directed to the injury site early to help plug the bleed. The plaques formed are then overgrown by normal cells and when these plaques are examined they are found to contain LDL, often in layers that represents repeated injury and healing as an ongoing process, like the rings in a tree.

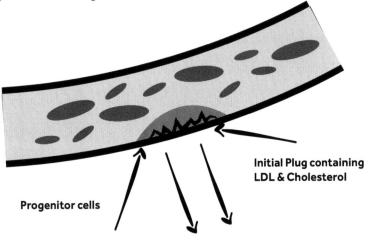

Initial Plug containing LDL & Cholesterol

Progenitor cells

An analogy will help to understand why cholesterol is always there at trouble sites. If there is a riot in town the police are called, they attend the scene and control the situation. If there is a road accident, the police attend the scene and resolve the situation. Similarly with a street fight the police attend the scene and calm the situation. Do the police cause these problems just because they are present at every incident?

Also if the police are removed will the riots and road accidents go away?

In the same way cholesterol is found at all these problem sites in the body but its role is positive not negative. If the problem had not been there in the first place, cholesterol plaques would not be found at that site.

Statins

If the "high fat diet increases cholesterol levels and clogs arteries" theory is pursued, thereby suggesting cholesterol as the cause of heart disease, which is currently the number one killer in the western world, then that creates an exciting opportunity for money to be made by anyone who could break into that chain of events. The food companies very quickly addressed every aspect of the diet angle and made fortunes out of convincing everyone to eat low-fat food substitutes. Now all that remained was for the drug companies to come up with a way of preventing the body from producing cholesterol at all and in theory that would solve the heart disease epidemic.

Possibly correct in principle but for the result to be positive, the theory must be correct in the first place and it is not!

Just spend a few minutes recapping from the list on an earlier page listing the invaluable role cholesterol plays in the body processes and then consider whether it is smart to prevent the body making it. Running with the diet/heart hypothesis, the drug companies tried to discover a drug to break the cholesterol production pathway. In the 14-step chemical conversion pathway required to produce cholesterol, there was only one chemical reaction that could be intercepted with a drug and safely halt cholesterol production at source. Interfering with any of the other 13 steps resulted in the death of the rats and rabbits used in the trials.

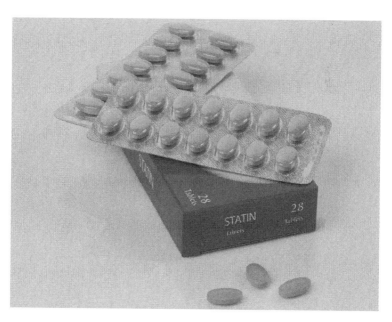

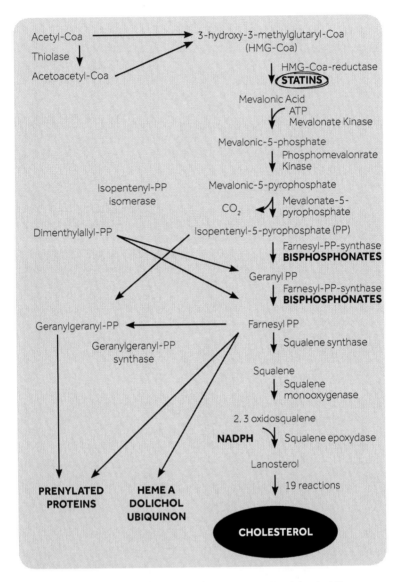

Statins do indeed lower cholesterol levels; they do indeed do what they say BUT they will not prolong life. You will die on the same day you were always destined to but you will die with lower cholesterol levels and all the side effects of living with lowered cholesterol levels.

That statement is alarming but it is true. Every long-term, large research study done into the use of statin drugs will claim ONLY to lower cholesterol levels. NOT ONE has EVER produced statistics on mortality rates. Many drug companies actively hide or refuse to publish mortality results. Why? Because they show statins making NO difference. Surely the only reason anyone would take a toxic drug with such horrible side effects is in the faith that it will prolong life? The side effects from statin use are reported in up to 40 per cent of cases and include abdominal pain, muscle or joint pain, muscle weakness, nerve injuries, memory loss, liver irritation and in severe cases have caused death by acute muscle degeneration or liver toxicity.

You may even have experienced the muscle issues associated with statin use and wondered why a drug for cholesterol lowering is so negatively affecting the muscles throughout the body. This side effect is a classic example of the dangers of not restoring balance within a body but overriding one system with a chemical and not bothering to understand the importance of cholesterol on other body functions. The knock-on effect of denying the body cholesterol is devastating. Every process that cholesterol is used for in the body slows or stops when statins are taken and that cannot happen without an impact on the normal function of the human body. One major problem is the dosage that is given; which is definitely a case of overkill. The desired effect of lower blood cholesterol can be reached on much lower doses than are often given. It is not uncommon to be on 40mg-plus a day when 5-10mg would be as beneficial without the toxic overload.

There is currently an incredible pressure to get cholesterol levels as low as possible and this helps fuel the overkill approach to dosage. This is particularly true for women, who in fact show NO correlation at all between dietary intake of fat, lowering cholesterol levels with statins and prevention of heart disease. Not one study has ever shown any benefit of statin use in women in preventing heart disease. There is one group who does show a helpful effect from taking statin drugs, although this is for reasons other than lowering cholesterol levels. Men who have already experienced a heart attack or coronary incident do decrease their chances of a second incident by taking statins. If you find yourself on statins you may like to consider taking Coenzyme Q10 to protect your cells from the damaging effect of the statin drug.

What REALLY causes heart disease?

The answer is well known, what is not really known or understood is exactly how the process becomes so devastating on the human body. That STRESS is the cause of heart disease (and many other chronic health diseases of the modern world) will probably not be a surprise but it may not be easy to really understand the true implications of what that means.

The human body is being forced to adapt to stress within its environment every econd of every day, and these stressors come constantly at all levels of our chemical, physical and emotional being.

How we choose to eat, move and think will have an impact our own internal stress response every second of every day. Learning how to control this will save your life. Knowing what causes the problem is only half the battle; solving it is the other. The solution does not lie in removing cholesterol from the body. Learning how to get off your iceberg will solve your problem.

We need cholesterol – without it we will die

We don't need stress – with it we will die

What's the answer?

As with all things concerning our health, the question is not "what do I take or do to treat the symptom but how do I address the cause?" The answer with heart disease is to live to reduce your stress.

Key factors have been PROVEN to help reduce heart disease:

Eating fruit and veg daily, raw if possible – this provides the body with essential nutrients. Enzymes cannot survive the cooking process and yet are essential to good health, so raw food is important to maintain a good supply of enzymes.

Exercise – this must be done daily for at least 30 minutes. It is important that the heart rate is increased by the exercise. Interval training is very beneficial.

Moderate consumption of wine – most people love reading this one! I emphasise this is NOT compulsory however there are good evidence based research documents that show truth in this.

The reason behind it is the relaxing effect one glass of wine can have within the body systems and the toxic effect is easily balanced out if the rest of the diet is good, hydration is high and exercise regime positive- balance in all things!

Omega 3 has proven benefits to the health of every cell in the body. It is viewed as an essential nutrient and is lacking in most western diets. It has a powerful effect in lowering raised cholesterol levels and should be considered an essential nutrient to maintain normal cholesterol levels or combat high ones. Source your supply carefully, quality is everything. When sourcing a supplement the rules are simple. You need to source one that has been molecularly distilled and consume it in a liquid form. The oil should NEVER smell fishy, if it does it has oxidised and will not benefit you.

Vitamin C should be provided daily to the human body. As a species we are incapable of making Vitamin C (only humans and a few species of monkeys cannot synthesise it!). The best source of this is fresh organic fruit and veg. However if this cannot be eaten a supplement should be taken. It will never offer as good a result but will improve the Vitamin C levels in the body. A word of caution; Vitamin C shares a receptor on a cell that is almost identical to glucose. If you have a high sugar diet it is very hard to get your body to use the vitamin C you provide it with as the receptors are all full up with glucose. Simply address your processed carbohydrate intake to solve this issue.

Anything you can do to manage your stress levels is helpful. Talking to friends, meditating, sourcing professional help, creating a community of supportive people around you is extremely beneficial to your wellbeing. Woman are very good at this but men are much less likely to find a support network and very much less likely to discuss concerns openly. This is known to have a serious impact on their stress levels. So, connect with your feminine side and learn to talk about your concerns and worries, it can save your life! (but just do what you are comfortable with, doing what other people expect you to do can be a stress in itself)

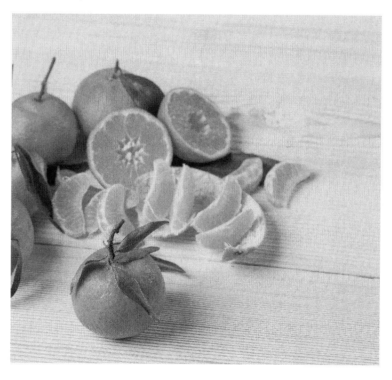

The most relevant causes of heart disease are:

1. High blood sugar levels, especially ones that spike

2. High insulin levels

3. Acute mental stress

4. Smoking

5. Cocaine use

6. Presence of Cortisol (stress hormone)

7. High levels of adrenalin

Alarm signals to watch out for are not your cholesterol levels but your waist measurement. As soon as you start storing fat around your organs (visceral fat), you have an important sign that you are in trouble.

If you are unlucky enough not to have been able to address lifestyle issues before a heart disorder begins then it is worth knowing that the best treatments available are drugs that have an effect on breaking down clots.

The PROVEN best treatments are any drug that breaks down clots or acts as an anticoagulant. Interestingly enough, one of the lesser-known or exploited uses of statins are their anti-coagulant affect. That is why men with a previous history of clots and heart disease can benefit from their use, NOT because it lowers their cholesterol but because it dissolves their clots.

In summary...

Changing your physical, emotional and chemical stressors will save your life.

For more information the book, 'The Great Cholesterol Con' by Dr Malcolm Kendrick is extremely useful it is humorous, sarcastic in places, a bit heavy-going at times but an absolute eye-opener in relation to the research that is out there on this subject and an absolute must-read for anyone with concerns about their own or a family member's risk of heart disease.

CHAPTER 8

CANCER

This is a massive topic and as the incidence of cancer rises, it is touching more and more lives. Even if you have not been touched personally it's certain that you will know someone that has received this devastating diagnosis. Because of the fear that surrounds this disease, it is one of the most dreaded diagnoses to receive. This chapter will try to address some of the positive steps that have been made towards understanding and treating cancer and offer some hope and understanding to those it affects.

Cancer affects one in three people and it is estimated that that statistic will change to one in two over the next ten years and beyond. That in itself is terrifying and explains why so much fear surrounds the disease. Even from childhood, most people will have been aware of the money that is poured into cancer research. In the 1970's there was a strong belief that the cause would be identified and both preventative measures and treatment regimes developed to save lives within just a few years. Whilst progress has been made, the numbers do not lie and the harsh truth is that what has been done so far really has not changed the course of this mega-killer. Science has studied and assessed, tested and diagnosed, treated and allowed experimental trials on people decade after decade, building up more and more data on the number of people diagnosed, their age, their occupation, their family history etc etc, yet the one thing that is not done is to focus on the two in every three people who DO NOT get cancer and ask the question - why do they NOT have cancer?

What have they done so differently? If the focus could be changed and health were studied, there would be a better chance of watching these statistics change, and in the next 10 years, seeing the numbers change to maybe one in four, then hopefully one in five as more people began duplicating lifestyles that match those that do not develop cancer and consequently prevent themselves developing this devastating disease.

Think about it for a moment, two in three people do NOT develop cancer. This group of people should be studied to find out why. I am sure we would all like to do everything in our power to make sure that we are in that group and if that means living our lives slightly differently, then I am happy with that. To never hear the words "I'm sorry to tell you but the tests have confirmed you have cancer" has to be worth some small lifestyle changes.

The evidence is there. People have beaten the most advanced cancers, they have put themselves into permanent remission and many more have lived lives that aim to ensure they never develop it in the first place.

When it comes to lifestyle changes, the most motivated group of people are those with a diagnosed illness. It is obvious why, they are staring down the barrel of a gun and want to change something; they are prepared to do anything to change their outcome. The challenge is when you appear symptom-free, you have no scary diagnosis to motivate you. How in that situation do you motivate yourself to do enough to prevent illness? That is a question only you can answer. At the beginning of this book, I discussed my fear of ageing and the realisation that it was not ageing per se that I feared most, but rather it was ageing with ill-health. Once we accept that we have control over our day-to-day decisions, we can choose to live to prevent illness. Taking back this power makes all the difference. We all have to die of something but we can live our lives determined to improve our chances and not sabotage our own health with poor choices each day.

It is known that cancer is essentially an immune system failure that allows mutated cells to take hold and multiply. Although the following fact may surprise and shock you, understanding the truth about the disease will help you make the right choices in how you live your life. Fact - we all have millions of cancer cells in us each and every day - they are mutated cells, not fit for purpose.

When the body's immune system is healthy these mutated cells are killed off instantly, they never take hold and settle into our tissues and we remain cancer-free If, however, our immune system is compromised, it is not strong enough to protect and defend us and these mutated cells begin to take over.

There is much talk about the genetic link to cancers, implying you have a blueprint in your genes for cancer and that would imply that you will develop cancer and there is nothing you can do about it. The argument against this theory is simple - no species on earth has ever had wired into its genetic makeup a blueprint for its own destruction. Cancer is a disease of our time. Its incidence has risen decade on decade for the last 50 years and yet our genes are the same as they have been for the last 10,000 years or more. Put simply, our genes have not changed. Something else is causing the rise in the incidence of cancer.

Sometimes there do appear to be very strong family links to cancer and it would seem that the writing is on the wall for some people. This, however, - coming from the DNA blueprint of their genes but is more likely coming from their environment. Families frequently live very similar lives, they eat the same foods, live in the same house, live through - and are susceptible to - the same stresses. Even though two people's lives are never identical, families provide more evidence of similar environmental exposure than any other demographic. The study of the environmental effects on our cells and genetic make-up is the science of epigenetics and this is an area of real excitement in the understanding of cancer.

Cancer cells need two things to be viable. Firstly, they need to be present because the immune system has not killed them off, and secondly they need a promoter to accelerate their growth and create the perfect environment where the body is weakened and the tumour can develop. The best example of this is smoking.

Cigarettes cause cancer - it is a known fact, it is written on every packet and science has proved this beyond doubt. In this scenario the cigarettes are the promoter, they suppress the immune system, pour toxic chemicals into the body, interfere with lung function and oxygen exchange and create the perfect environment for mutated cells that should have been killed off, to take hold and grow.

If you smoke you will develop lung cancer - guaranteed - what varies for people is the time frame required to develop the cancer. In some people that is a matter of just a few years, others may die of something else before the cancer kills them. It is certain that if everyone who smoked lived long enough, every single person would develop cancer - no exceptions. That is why on every packet of cigarettes they can legally state that smoking kills, smoking causes cancer. It is simply because science has now proved beyond any doubt that it is the only outcome for smokers. An individual may just have needed to be 120 years old to develop it! So, when you meet someone who tells you they smoked for 60 years and never got cancer, the answer is they just have not yet lived long enough to develop the cancer.

Once you can understand that the environment your body finds itself in is what dictates the ability of a cancer cell to take hold, you can see that YOU actually hold the power, you can make decisions each day to live a cleaner, safer life. Studying the people who do not develop cancer makes so much sense because by copying their lifestyles and adopting their habits, you put yourself on a health curve instead of a sickness curve. Let us live to prevent cancer because that takes away the fear of ever being diagnosed with it.

The immune system is absolutely key here. If your immune system is fully functional, you never have to worry about cancer. If, however, your immune system is under stress and not fully functional, then your chances of cancer cells not being killed off increases. So the greatest support I can offer you is to highlight some of the things that have a negative impact on your immune systems; you may be surprised to learn that they can start as early as when you are first born.

Seventy percent of your immune system comes from your bowel bacteria. This was touched on in an earlier chapter but it is necessary to revisit here and show how relevant to cancer prevention it is. The very first dose of bowel bacteria a baby gets is from its mother as it is born. Sterile deliveries and C-sections have a serious impact on this first dose of bacteria passing to the baby. The bowel health of the mother is also extremely relevant, if she has little or no healthy bowel bacteria, there is nothing good to pass on.

Assuming that process did happen and all is well, the next problem encountered may be the type of milk the baby is fed; breast milk is most certainly best when it comes to antibodies and growing a healthy bowel flora, nothing balances pH better and is more digestible to a newborn than human breast milk. Formula milk is now packed with high- fructose corn syrup and dairy protein molecules that are large and can be irritating to the bowels. The high sugar content from corn syrup creates an imbalance in bowel bacteria where the bacteria that love an acidic environment thrive and those that seek the healthier alkaline environment die off.

The next hit comes from vaccinations. At eight weeks old a vaccination programme is started in most countries, especially those in the developed Western world. At this young age, the immature immune system is ill equipped to cope with a hit every few weeks of multiple killer diseases. This book is not the place to discuss the whole issue of vaccination but there is no denying that the immune system is extremely immature in these early weeks and the constant exposure to this intense immunisation programme has the potential to adversely affect the developing immune system in a broad and long-term way.

Another major issue is any antibiotic medication that is given to a child - this wipes out the bowel bacteria in the process of wiping out the infection and the legacy of that can be very far reaching.

Diet is another major area of concern. If an acidic environment is created internally, the result is a prolific overgrowth of 'bad' bacteria, this leads to the suppression of other bacteria and the balance of the bowel flora is altered. Our food choices dictate our internal pH. For children, the most acidic foods are grains, dairy, soy, meat, sugars and sweet drinks, for adults you can add coffee, tea and alcohol as key culprits.

One of the biggest triggers to suppression of the immune system is stress which can be physical, emotional or chemical. Whichever angle it comes at you from, the outcome is exactly the same, the immune system is shut down. The reason for this is very simple - when we are stressed the body has a pre-programmed chemical response, it releases cortisol and adrenalin and goes into the flight or fight response. This puts activity within the immune system on hold for as long as you remain in the flight or fight response. A short- term stress response when in survival mode is perfectly acceptable. However, long-term existence within that flight or fight scenario is extremely detrimental. Continuing in stress mode for days, weeks or months is a recipe for disaster.

As you will appreciate from this brief summary of our first few months of life and the common trap of living life with chronic stress, an acidic internal environment and poor bowel flora, there are pitfalls to navigate to ensure we give ourselves the best chance at developing and maintaining a strong immune system.

If you are reading this and feeling panicked that you have a poor immune system and that you have raised children that most likely also have a poor immune system, then please be reassured that these things can be reversed. You can build a healthy bowel flora again, restore a fully functioning immune system and live a lifestyle that promotes health within these systems.

Fermented foods or supplementation with pre and probiotics are the absolute best ways to do this and depending on the age you are when wanting to make these improvements depends very much on the approach that needs to be taken.

It should go without saying, that removing the stress in your life, getting off your iceberg, is imperative and should be a priority. Hopefully, reading through this book has shown you where the imbalances and stressors can be coming from.

The topic of bowel flora was covered in detail earlier in this book and you may find it helpful to review that section and also the acid/alkaline diet if you are keen to correct the balance in your digestive system. You will find practical advice at the back of this book to help you navigate your way through these changes.

One very interesting link and one that is not that obvious on the surface, is the correlation between exercise and the decreased occurrence of cancer.

Some quite remarkable statistics are available showing the phenomenal impact of regular exercise on all types of cancers, whether they be hormone-promoted, site specific or metastases. You may be wondering how is this even possible? How does a brisk 30-minute walk each day decrease your chance of developing colon cancer by 50%, or your chance of lung cancer by more than 70%? The best way to understand the answers to this is to revisit the basics and look again at the three areas of stress we all live with - how we move, eat and think.

You can be deficient in good healthy activity. If you sit more than three hours a day you are literally toxic with too much sitting, and deficient in healthy activity. We know this because, historically, human beings moved for hours every day, they moved through their days lifting, carrying, pushing, pulling, walking and running. Modern-day living looks nothing like the life we are blueprinted to lead, we are not programmed to sit for hours and hours each day, we are programmed for movement, for our genetic makeup derives from an era about 10,000 years ago, so whatever we were eating, thinking or however we were moving at that time, is the blueprint for our health, even today. Until our genetic blueprint goes through a massive evolution to create the next "form" of human being, we have to accept this is true. If we can take some of the rules from way back and apply them to our modern-day lives, we have a framework to build lives that are healthier than the ones we are living.

Toxicity and deficiency lie behind every chronic illness and we can reclaim the power of our own health by working to correct the deficiency and remove the toxicity.

When any stress presents itself to the body it launches the stress response, which is the only way we change our physiology and have a chance of surviving the stress we face at that moment. The chemistry within us that we create with the stress reaction is to enable us to either fight or flee. Both of these are physical activities and both result in a lowering of adrenalin and cortisol in the bloodstream and an increase in serotonin (happy hormone). The end result of that response is the immune system is able to function again, rather than being placed on "hold" as it is during the stress response.

That in a nutshell is why cancer rates can be reduced with exercise. We switch our immune response back on when we address the cause which is stress - physical, chemical or emotional or probably a combination of all three! The solution for each is exercise.

This system is so well designed that even if the stress is chemical or emotional, the physical act of doing exercise has the same effect. It breaks the cycle of suspended function of the immune system and allows it to work again.

The key to success with this approach is regular exercise, to be consistently committed to a physical pursuit, hopefully something you enjoy. To schedule time to do it and to prioritise it as if your life depends on it, because it quite literally does! If you are making excuses to not exercise, it is probably because you don't realise how important it is when considering your health. It's so much more than a toned, muscular body; it goes to the very core of your wellbeing and the prevention of chronic illness.

The last point to cover is 'self-talk' and emotional stress and how that can be linked to cancer. Emotional stress can be real or imagined, which means you can find yourself in a very real situation that has you emotionally challenged and stressed, that is usually based on real fear. As a result, you push yourself physiologically into the stress response. Physical exercise can help with this type of stress, go for a run or a brisk walk and you will feel better able to deal with the issue at hand. Be it a stressful day at work, deadlines, a grumpy boss, work colleagues and office politics, all very real and very stressful. You will find going for a brisk walk at lunchtime will lower your personal stress levels and make you better able to cope with the situation in front of you and internally you will be managing your adrenalin levels and helping maintain balance within your body.

Then there is imagined emotional stress, where your thoughts run away with you and you can upset yourself over a situation that has not yet happened, may never happen and yet you worry yourself into the stress response. You experience anxiety and fear over something not real and very often something you can do nothing about. You develop stories and scenarios in your head that quite simply are made up!

Luckily for us, the same solution exists, physical exercise will decrease the response. This goes back to the basic principles of the flight or fight response, both require a physical outlay of energy to change the body's chemistry.

There are also many mind-control techniques that you can use to control your anxiety. One very simple and effective one is based around visualisation of a positive outcome. Think past your current concern and fear and imagine an outcome that just means the thing you are worrying about cannot possibly happen.

When I first heard this example from Mel Robbins in her book The 5 Second Rule, I realised the power we hold over our imagined fears and anxieties, so I'm sharing it with you here and hope it helps you too, with a simple technique for taking back control of your thoughts.

Imagine you have a fear a flying, making you worry every second you are on the plane, it can be perfectly smooth with no problems and yet you are convincing yourself it is going to drop out the sky any second and you will never see your family again! To take back control, you need to change the image in your mind from one that involves the plane crashing to one where all is well, you have not crashed to the ground and you are safe. So your visualisation may include something like walking in your front door and being greeted by your family, then going out to your favourite restaurant for dinner, because obviously if that is what your brain is seeing as your reality the plane did not crash and you are fine. It is a mind game, but it works really well. Change your end result with a strong, positive image and you will decrease your anxiety. Preferably use an image with emotion attached, like the hug of a greeting from you children, or the smell and taste of your favourite meal in the restaurant. Make it real by attaching feelings to your visualisation.

This technique works best when you have thought beforehand what your positive visualisation is going to be, if you try and work all this out while you are fearful and anxious it will not work.

One last point about 'self-talk'; please, please, please be aware of and careful about what you are telling yourself, if you talk to yourself in a negative, unloving, unsupportive way, you will create stress within yourself. Specifically, you may have a very negative thought pattern based around your fear of developing cancer, you may tell yourself daily that your mother had it therefore you will inevitably develop it, too. This HAS to STOP! It is not real and it creates imagined fear and stress, based in nothing but an incorrect story you are telling yourself. Change the story! It will save your life.

Keep telling yourself the same story and you will get what you are telling yourself in the story. The mind cannot differentiate between real and imagined. The sporting world is capitalising on this and teaching sports professionals how to visualise the win before they are even in the game. The genius of this technique is it really works. The mind attracts the outcome it thinks about.

The power of attraction works for both good and bad things, make sure you attract health not sickness.

Hopefully, this chapter has made you feel you can win back some control of your destiny and start to understand it is not predetermined, you are not a ticking time-bomb, you have the ability to live the life that either will or will not lead to cancer. The choice is yours.

A Story About Taking Control Back

Being told out of the blue that I had cancer was the greatest shock of my life. The feeling of numbness and confusion is hard to describe. It's like a bereavement. All I could think and say whilst crying helplessly at the GP was; I haven't got time to be ill!! How can I have cancer?

The weeks that followed are all a blur as I was I in a state of shock. I remember crumbling in the doctors office just screaming that I don't want to die. It's a feeling you don't wish on anyone, sort of an empty terrifying feeling of unfair helplessness. I couldn't say the word Cancer for many weeks, let alone accepting that I had it. Often I used to find myself forgetting I had cancer and then like I had woken up from a nightmare I would remember I did. The moments when I forgot never lasted more than a few seconds.

When you have cancer you are supposed to look after yourself first and foremost. I can't do that though. My 16 year old daughter has been very ill since early autumn of 2018 with chronic pain and I was caring for her 24/7 when I was diagnosed with cancer. I was also researching what was wrong with her and trying to find someone who could help her as no doctor seemed to have any idea. I often wonder how life can be this cruel yet somehow you have to deal with what you are given, no matter how difficult. The day I was given the diagnose I was supposed to book plane tickets to take my daughter to the USA in January for medical treatment. Instead I had to tell my family I had cancer and that my daughter's potential road to recovery had to be delayed. The cruellest thing possible which goes against everything I believe in or who I am.

I went through various scans and tests and a date for surgery was set to remove the tumour on my ovary and hopefully as many lymph nodes as possible. By now I could say the word cancer and started to feel I needed to try to take charge of the cancer instead of the cancer taking charge of me. This is when I contacted Debbie who I knew believes in taking care of your body as the key to health. She advised me what types of food feed the cancer and what foods to eat to try to help me beat the cancer. I found this extremely helpful as it gave me power. This is my way of taking charge of my situation as no doctor will advice on any diet. I have not touched a drop of alcohol either since my diagnosis as I don't want to put my body under unnecessary stress. I have stuck with the diet advice Debbie gave me apart from a few small glitches!

Being on a strict diet isn't always easy but I just have to remind myself now and then why I'm doing it. I'm doing it for me, to try to help my body to heal and fight cancer. I will do anything to beat this beast.

After my 4th round of chemo I had a CT scan to see if the cancer was spreading or shrinking. Yesterday I got the results and I am happy to share that my cancer is shrinking and the large tumour on a large blood vessel they couldn't remove during surgery is also shrinking. I am a firm believer that I have helped to get to this point with the power of food and following Debbie's diet advice. Some might say it wouldn't have made any difference. There is no way of telling, but I know my cancer is shrinking and it's on its way out of my body. I am also feeling much better in myself despite having gruelling chemotherapy. Even the consultant commented on how well I look for someone who's had 4 chemotherapy treatments and is as seriously ill as I actually am.

I still have a long way to go until I am cancer free, but the power of foods is amazing. I am not ready to let this beast beat me, my children are still young and I am definitely not ready to leave them for many years. Living with cancer is a very scary place but with a strong mind, determination and the right food and medical treatment I will beat it!

Ylva's Story

CHAPTER 9
Alzheimer's and Dementia

Over the last 10 years the incidence of this disease has risen, although not as much as was predicted. This fact may surprise you as so many people are affected either directly or indirectly by this devastating condition but the perception of its rise in incidence is due to the current rising population of over 60's. This is great news and means we are probably doing something right and changing the course of the disease, albeit very slowly, and against the fact of a large and increasing demographic of people in the over 60's category.

Dementia in all its forms, has its strongest link to age as the causal factor, with an incidence of just a few per hundred aged 65-69, yet by the mid-eighties this has risen to one in five (20 per cent). Stopping the ageing process is impossible but there are lifestyles which can be adopted that will help our brain cells stay healthy, and these are simple things that we can all do.

Luckily, these are the same things that help to combat so many other chronic diseases so it becomes a matter of putting in the work once and reaping the benefits over and over in the many systems of our bodies.

Here is a recap of the direct things you can do to lower your risk of dementia.

- do not smoke
- exercise daily - 30 minutes of a brisk walk is enough
- eat to nourish your body
- keep your toxic load as low as possible
- maintain a healthy blood pressure
- maintain a healthy weight and be mindful of your waist measurement
- drink alcohol according to guidelines or preferably not at all

Smoking and drinking literally kill off your brain cells. Both deliver chemicals into your bloodstream that cross the blood brain barrier and cell death is the consequence. If you choose to smoke or drink consistently for a period of time, you will increase your risk of early onset dementia, your brain cells will die off faster than they can regenerate when under a constant toxic load from these sources.

Exercise stimulates the nervous system and is well known to have a huge benefit to the body's general wellbeing; whether that be weight, blood pressure, stress, cholesterol levels, blood glucose levels etc. When considering exercise in your lifestyle, do not think of running a marathon, what seems to impact health most is consistent activity that increases the heart and breathing rates for 30 minutes, five times a week. So keep it simple and aim for a brisk 30-minute walk each day to gain all these benefits.

If you have ever sat at your desk feeling brain-dead and sluggish, then got up, moved your body and been able to go back and do desk work again feeling revived, THAT is the effect of exercise on stimulating the nervous system. We should utilise it to get optimum productivity in the classroom and workplace, if you move around you are smarter than when you sit still!

Nourishing your body with great nutrition is important on every level, every function in your body relies on fuel, chemicals and communication. The brain function creates a huge demand for fats and knowing which fats are good for us and which are not is important. The earlier chapter on cholesterol will, I hope, have helped you to understand this topic. Essential fatty acids, particularly Omega 3 are super important for our brains as well as a substance called phosphatidylserine, another fatty substance known as a phospholipid, which is receiving a lot of attention currently as an essential nutrient to protect and restore brain cell health. It is primarily found in meat-based products, however, there are plant-based sources of it such as soy beans, white beans, cabbage, carrots, whole-grain barley, and rice.

Eat foods filled with healthy fats such as avocados, coconut oil, olive oil and supplement high quality omega 3's and phosphtidylserine and you will have a diet that is providing your brain with the essential nutrients it needs. The brain is 70% cholesterol and fats and if you lower your fat intake, you risk removing the food source that keeps it healthy. Choose your fats carefully and always choose to eat them daily.

Ensuring a sufficiency of nutrients to maintain health is only half the picture, you must also lower the toxins that damage your brain cells. Although I have touched on smoking and alcohol consumption, there are other factors that should be considered. The most serious of these and the one you should be most aware of is heavy metals - particularly mercury and lead.

Heavy metals have a real affinity for the brain, which acts like a magnet and attracts these toxic agents and once there, they stay and wreak havoc. Cell death and neurological disruption are common when levels of heavy metal exposure exist. Some of your exposure to these metals will be historical but there are some current areas of risk.

Growing up with lead pipes for plumbing will have have produced quite a build-up within your system. Every drink you every took and very bath you ever had will have delivered some lead into your system which never leaves and is stored in the nervous system, primarily your brain.

- If you use lipstick that contains lead you are ingesting that daily

- If you work directly with metals you will inhale vapours and absorb product though your skin

- If you have every had an amalgam filling you have mercury in your mouth, combined with other metals such as silver, tin and copper amalgam fillings have been used for decades and controversy surrounds them and associated health issues. Elemental mercury can leach from the fillings and pass into the digestive system as can small sections of a filling as they degrade. Mercury can be absorbed as vapour from leaking fillings. These are known to be linked to allergic reactions, skin and gum disorders and digestive issues. Accumulation of mercury as a toxin occurs most highly in the kidneys and nervous system. If two fillings contact each other when you bite they will ultimately break down and release both vapours and material into your digestive system, which then works its way around your body to settle in your tissues and organs.

- Many fillings are now made of composite, a material based in a resin, they offer a great colour match to a tooth, yet many contain BPA and other toxins found in plastic resins. Alternatives and BPA-free composites are available if you ask you dentist.

- Vaccinations historically contained thimerosal, a mercury-based stabiliser that was injected directly into your body with each vaccine. Realising that mercury within the blood system was not ideal, vaccinations swapped from that practise and the adjuvant now used is aluminium. It could be argued this is not much of an improvement, as this is a relatively new practise and the links to Alzheimer's have not been eliminated or confirmed.

- Glyphosate, better known as Roundup is a chemical herbicide that acts like an antibiotic, destroying healthy flora in plants and in ourselves. Once this water-soluble substance enters our bodies, it causes the breakdown of protective membranes and you see conditions such as leaky gut, sinus issues, dementia, heart and blood pressure issues. Specifically avoid the following items as they contain overly-high residue amounts of glyphosate:

  • Soya (this means soya products and soya or vegetable oil)

  • Corn and corn oil

  • Canola seeds used in canola oil

- Beets and beet sugar
- Almonds
- Dried peas
- Carrots
- Quinoa
- Sweet potatoes

It is advisable to buy organic fruits and vegetable whenever possible as washing alone will not remove this toxic chemical as it works its way into the flesh of the food it touches.

This is true for meat also as the animals are often given feeds that are toxic with glyphosate and it will accumulate in the fat and skin of that animal. This is always best removed before eating and to be absolutely sure it is best to buy organic, grass-fed meats.

- Lastly, let's revisit sweeteners and remind ourselves of the cell damage they cause when they cross the blood brain barrier and cause neuroexcitation, where the cells quite literally vibrate themselves to death.

Applying other good lifestyle practises, such as maintaining a healthy weight, healthy blood pressure and well maintained blood-glucose levels will go a long way towards keeping your brain active, functioning and renewing cells.

Many people benefit from keeping their minds active on a daily basis by taking the time to exercise their brains with crosswords, quizzes, Sudoko and other mind games. Think of it a little like going to the gym for your brain!

This is not a huge chapter for the simple reason that living by the Complete Lifestyle principles of supplying sufficiency and removing toxicity will keep both your body healthy and your brain functioning. Add in the specific nutrients necessary for brain health and cut out the specific toxins that damage our brains and you will go a long way to being as bright as a button for 90-years-plus!

If you are a carer for someone with dementia or Alzheimer's, you will be under the most enormous strain. Shock, fear, loneliness and grief are just some of the daily emotions you will find yourself having to cope with. The stress load you carry daily would, for most people, seem unbearable, but the stress load you carry will build silently each day, loading you more and more over the years, without you even realising quite how severe the stress load you are carrying is. This will affect YOUR health. This is your personal iceberg and although you know you cannot get off it, I would implore you to try and find a way to think about yourself and work where you can to decrease your stress-load. Diet is an excellent way to do this, keep putting in great nutrition and removing toxins with each meal choice you make, you will find this benefits your energy, your immune system, your ability to cope, your sleep patterns and your digestive system.

Because you are constantly in the stress response of flight or fight, you will find huge benefit from physical exercise, raising your heart rate 3-5 times a week with 20-30 minutes of exercise will always decrease the amount of adrenalin in your system and slow the onset of adrenal fatigue which, once it occurs, can leave you trying to run on empty in a situation you know you need to be in top shape to survive.

The wake of devastation this disease leaves is unique as both the physical and emotional assault continues over such a prolonged period and affects all parties in different ways. Learning to accept help in whatever format it is offered can develop lifelines of coping strategies that help you get through each day. Ask for help, accept help and please give yourself a thought in amongst the heartbreak and stress of your role as a carer.

The Long Journey Back from Stress

When my husband was diagnosed with dementia it confirmed what I had known for a couple of years, despite the mental health service telling me repeatedly that he had "at worst some cognitive impairment".

The illness was retrospectively diagnosed as having probably begun in 2007. In 2011 my husband's behaviour was very dysfunctional , diagnosis was in October 2014 and by 23rd Dec 2017 he was dead.

I have never done anything harder in my 63 years than care for my husband during that three year period.

My husband John was a big, strong, fit sportsman, he played rugby for his city, county and country, he was handsome, well dressed and always smelled delicious. In a three year period the things I loved and that made him him were stripped away.

I remember a member of the mental health team visiting us just after diagnosis and telling me I couldn't manage this on my own.

I felt duty bound to prove her wrong , he was my husband, I loved him, it was my role to care for him, nobody else's.

Fortunately this lady wouldn't take no for an answer and despite my reluctance, organised for John to attend a day club for 5 hours once a week.

That short respite allowed me a break from the illness and as he worsened so our dependence on the day club grew.

Nothing in my life had prepared me for the the descent into Alzheimers. I could not and still cannot understand how someone else's illness has had such an effect on my health. I remember thinking, if this is how I feel at 60, what must it be like if you're 70 or 80 and having to care for a loved one with this terrible condition. The physicality required is inestimable, the mental strain and drain even worse.

Repeatedly I was told that I couldn't care for him if I didn't first care for myself but I had neither the will nor the wherewithal to do more than fight my way through each day, trying to ensure John had what he needed to be as well and happy as possible.

I learned there is a huge void between what support is promised and what actually exists, the system is at best broken, if not non existent.

If I had to sum up my journey I would liken myself to the little crab popped into a pan of cold water and then brought to the boil, oblivious to the fact of being broiled to death.

Seventeen months after my husbands death my body is unable to let go of the stress. My doctor says that once learned the body finds it very hard to let go of this ingrained anxiety. Learning how to live without the anxiety again is going to be a long process yet it is something I am committed to.

I used to be mistaken for being 10 years younger than my age. In the space of three years that altered and I'm amazed that someone else's illness could have aged me visibly so much. The most devastating visual of the stress I was under was how it aged me.

I found it impossible to care for myself as well as my husband, my desire to love and keep him safe, to make his life as good as possible took all my time and effort.

It's now a year and a half since John died, finally I'm learning to look after myself. I found it impossible to find the time to do this when he was ill.

I would urge anyone caring to make a better job of looking after themselves than I managed. Ask for help, talk and reach out, eat well, sleep, rest and get fresh air and exercise. Don't be a crab.

And if you know someone who is caring then please step in and give them the space and support to be well themselves. Insist. It matters, it matters so much.

Carol and John's Story

CHAPTER 10

Raising Healthy Children in the Modern World

This is a very important sector of the book because children are our future! If you are battling stroppy teenagers or are sleep-deprived because of a screaming baby, you may not immediately share the sentiment behind that statement, but the truth is, that to evolve as a species, the human race needs to pass on its strengths and lose its weaknesses. Children watch us and learn from us, so it is our primary duty to do the best for them that we can and that starts with doing the best for ourselves. That means living a life that is the happiest, healthiest and strongest possible version of ourselves. Every generation will do things slightly differently, times will certainly change and, without doubt, we will evolve as a species. Ensuring that evolution is in the right direction is very much the basis of this book.

The aim of this section is to introduce you to the best health and lifestyle practises for different stages of a child's life; the part you can play in that and how, by applying some very simple principles, you can keep a growing child's body in a balanced state, free of toxins and nutritionally supplied with everything that is required for growth and repair.

Pre-Conceptive Care

If you are lucky enough to be able to plan your pregnancy, you have an incredible advantage as pre-conceptive care is invaluable in setting the health scene for your baby's life. This involves both mum and dad and takes about six months of dedicated effort, but the benefits are proven.

Coming off all contraceptive hormone treatments is number one. This means, for a few months, alternative contraceptive methods will need to be employed but it is important to get the synthetically produced hormones out of your body and allow a few months to restore normal hormone levels before you try to get pregnant.

All the sex hormones like oestrogen, progesterone and testosterone are steroid-based, which means they rely on cholesterol for their production. It is prudent to look closely at your diet and ensure enough cholesterol-forming foods are being eaten. Great sources of cholesterol are eggs, nuts and oils. Avoiding all low fat options for your food choices is helpful as these have had all the essential fats, the very fats that your body will now be looking for, removed. Take Omega 3 daily, about 1 teaspoon of high quality molecularly distilled oil will provide you with your daily requirement. Remember, quality is everything, good quality omega oils do not smell fishy in any way.

Essentially, the aim must be to decrease the total toxic load on your body in all three of the categories already discussed. Start by eating clean foods that will allow a rest period for your body and it will soon release toxins from their stored locations in the fat cells around your body.

Details of a recommended clean eating plan can be found on my website www.completelifestyle.co.uk

Enjoy eating the 'rainbow' and flooding your body with nutrients from fresh organic fruits and vegetables. This will provide the body with a sufficiency of vitamins and minerals. Eating these foods raw will also give the body a much-needed shot of vital enzymes. Enzymes are destroyed in the cooking process, hence the requirement for fruits and vegetables to be eaten raw to deliver a good supply of enzymes.

The building blocks for growth and repair come from protein and this is best obtained from sources such as nuts and pulses, vegan protein or high quality grass-fed organic meats that can guarantee no antibiotic or hormone use.

We require high-quality fats and this does not include margarine, soft spreads or vegetable oils, which are best avoided.

We need carbohydrates for energy in the form of fruits and vegetables not in the processed forms we are all so used to. If we are choosing grains they should to be organic whole grains, preferably brown rice, quinoa, millet, spelt, rye or barley not wheat.

Good items to remove from your diet are the addictive, allergenic and acidic foods such processed sugars, high fructose corn syrup and artificial sweeteners; these are the worst culprits and should be avoided at all costs. They are found in common foods such as fizzy drinks, diet foods, chewing gum and all sweets and biscuits.

The problem with dairy and processed grains are they make our internal pH very acidic and now is an excellent time to cut them down or out completely, alkalising your body creates balance in all its systems and that includes your hormone system. Use alternatives such as organic rice milk, coconut, almond or oat milk and changing your choice of meals and snacks away from the processed grains to healthy alternatives is a smart move.

It is essential to drink plenty of water - at least two litres a day and to avoid toxic drinks such as coffee, tea, alcohol and fizzy sodas, especially diet versions.

A good supplement routine includes daily omega 3, a good quality probiotic, greens powder and easily digestible protein.

This regime will provide your body with all it requires to be healthy and address the toxicity issue by cutting out toxic foods. Following this as closely as possible for as long as you can prior to trying to conceive your baby will achieve the required balance in your health and if this can be achieved in both parents, the perfect internal environment for the sperm and egg will be created.

There are terrifyingly high rates of infertility in westernised countries and it is no coincidence that our diets have become devoid of essential nutrients, highly acidic, allergenic and our bodies have shut down particular processes. Add to this the chemical imbalance created by hormone treatments such as contraception, the chronic stress we all live under - plus the toxic load of chemicals we are exposed to in our environment and that has produced a recipe for fertility disaster.

Remember, the body is programmed with an innate intelligence to be balanced and healthy. If your body is out of balance and you can remove interference and provide sufficiency, it will soon see improved function.

Exercise has an important role in wellbeing, so now might be the time to step up whatever physical activity you usually do. If nothing is your usual level, then it's time to get active! Aim for no less than 30 minutes a day. You need to support your heart and get your stress levels down and there is no better way to do that than through exercise. You may enjoy involving each other in exercise hobbies, all too soon there may be little feet around and the dynamics will change forever! Enjoy your free time together now but choose activities that benefit your health.

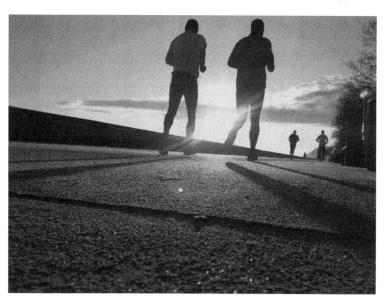

Finally, think about your emotional stress levels. If something is really adding to your stress load, address it now because when the baby comes along it will only increase the pressure. Spend some time talking together about your current position, jobs, houses, friends and family and discuss the dynamics that might not be working for you, consider changes and review options. Look to the future and check your current course is in line with that.

Babies come with a host of new, unfamiliar stressors and you need to have a tight handle on your current position to get through them easily.

This may seem like a lot of work but what you are actually doing is quickly teaching yourselves a new way to live. You are learning skills and life habits that you will use throughout the pregnancy and then be able to pass on to your baby. By living to decrease stressors on your body, you will live a much happier, healthier life. There is no greater reason to engage with this process than a plan to bring a baby into this world but it is actually something we should all do daily to improve our own wellbeing. You will be a great role model for your baby/child and have improved health, energy and vitality. Pregnancy is not a journey that a woman goes on alone, every man has an enormous supporting role and understanding just how important that role is, can make for a happier, healthier pregnancy.

Not all pregnancies have this type of planned lead up; some take us a little more by surprise! There is no need to panic if you have not been able to give your baby the best start, just begin as quickly as possible to make all the improvements listed above and your body will soon catch up. Your baby will take all it needs from you so if you're not 100% fit and healthy when you conceive you need not worry too much; your baby will be finding all it needs at your expense. The description above is of an ideal scenario where both the mother and father can be involved in the healthy preparation of a pregnancy.

CHAPTER 11
Pregnancy

Congratulations, you've made it this far! Only a lifetime to go!

There are two aspects to this part of your journey - what <u>you</u> need through the pregnancy and what <u>your baby</u> needs, although you are intrinsically linked and your baby will take what it needs from you, exactly when it needs it, at whatever cost to you. It is best to avoid getting into that situation and instead have a happy partnership where you are both sufficiently provided for.

What the baby needs

You may feel a real sense of wonder, you may even be feeling quite clever, after all you have got pregnant! But lesson number one in this whole miracle is that apart from supporting your body, nature has pretty well got this one worked out. Without interference your body will be able to produce for you in nine months a perfectly-formed baby. From two cells it can create a perfect little human. You can do some appalling things to yourself, through sickness or abuse and your baby will continue to grow and develop, maybe not to its maximum potential but it will develop. This is the power of the innate intelligence of the body, that with virtually no input from the mother, it can grow a baby. The real wonder of this process is quite amazing and extremely humbling.

When considering the baby's needs, the important thing to remember is that your baby is living symbiotically in you/with you and whatever is good for you, will be good for your baby, and whatever is bad for you will also be bad for your baby. The rules are simple; living up to them can sometimes be much harder.

The internal environment inside the womb is perfect for your baby and your detoxifying organs such as liver and kidneys, lungs and skin will be working hard to make sure nothing passes into that environment that would damage your baby. The placenta also plays an invaluable role in filtering out harmful substances. Sadly, some of the toxins we are now exposed to in the modern world can pass to the baby, cigarette smoke and alcohol are classic examples of harmful toxins that babies are all too frequently exposed to. Less well-known chemicals also enter the baby's world and have the potential to interfere with development. Examples of these include: chlorine and fluoride, pesticides such as glyphosate and heavy metals from mercury dental fillings and historically vaccinations. Skin creams and hygiene products are also packed with chemicals that pass directly into the blood stream, via the skin.

A baby's needs at this time are limited to requiring a toxin-free environment and a food supply that provides ALL essential nutrients. This is easier said than done, but on the plus- side, both you and your developing baby require the same nutrients. If you can look after yourself well and really put some effort into good dietary choices, your baby will be getting everything they require, too.

Omega 3 and probiotics are the nutrient supplements that I would advice taking daily, it could be argued that everything else can be obtained from a good diet, but sometimes supplementation is needed. Avoiding pesticides and herbicides means buying organic but that is a wise health choice for life, not just for pregnancy.

Your body will have an extra demand placed on it for folic acid, B vitamins, iron, vitamin C, calcium, magnesium, Vitamin K, E and zinc, water and calories in general.

Folic Acid

Your body needs double the amount of folic acid during pregnancy and current guidelines recommend taking it prior to conception to help build supplies. It is used in cell division within the DNA and RNA . Deficiency often presents as abnormalities in the skeleton such as spina bifida, heart, lungs, cleft lips, cleft palette, miscarriages and anaemia.

Folic acid is part of the B vitamin group and is therefore found in green, leafy vegetables. Wheatgrass (fresh or freeze-dried) represents an amazing source of B vitamins.

Iron

This is vital for haemoglobin production in red blood cells. The demand for this increases in pregnancy, as more oxygen carrying capacity is needed in the blood. Great food sources are dark green, leafy vegetables, seaweeds, lean meats (grass-fed, hormone-free) and high-quality fish, nuts and some beans and pulses.

Vitamin C

Human beings cannot synthesise vitamin C, and are entirely dependent on their diets for it. Vitamin C is needed to aid the absorption of iron and also for bone and tooth formation. It is common in many foods especially citrus foods and peppers. Try and eat your Vitamin C requirement from organic fruits and not chemically produced ascorbic acid supplements.

Calcium

Calcium is a mineral; it is needed for strong teeth and bones, but please don't confuse this statement with a need for dairy foods. This was discussed in detail in the chapter about Dairy and confusing these two truths has created a protracted belief that dairy provides human beings with the calcium they require. This is simply not the whole truth. Calcium is very important through pregnancy but not dairy products and especially not milk. Pasteurised milk represents a toxic food that delivers hormones, antibiotics, puss cells and zero natural nutrients (due to the pasteurisation process) it makes the internal environment of the human body acidic (it needs to be alkaline to be healthy.) Relying on dairy products as a stable part of a diet, in my opinion is a mistake. Research shows strong links between exposure to dairy products both in utero, and when newborn, and disorders such as eczema, asthma, diabetes and other allergic reactions.

Some good news about dairy – partially fermented yoghurt with no added sugar and some Swiss cheeses have high calcium levels and parmesan contains the highest levels of calcium in all cheeses. Butter contains butyric acid and high levels of vitamin A as well as Vitamins E, K and D, all essential for good health.

The cows we are milking to provide us with calcium are receiving their calcium through their diet - they are eating the plants that are rich in calcium, this is calcium absorbed from the ground. So, if we just cut out the middle cow and eat the plants ourselves we will get a much healthier version of calcium, one our bodies can actually utilise without negative reactions.

Our greatest source of useable calcium is organic vegetables especially green, leafy ones such as parsley, broccoli and spinach, so include plenty of these in your daily diet and you will do far better than by drinking a pint of cow's milk.

Magnesium

Magnesium is another essential mineral important for the correct function of nerves and muscles, it plays an important role in preventing miscarriage. Good food sources for magnesium are Brazil nuts, cashew nuts, almonds, sunflower seeds, hazelnuts, figs, seaweed, kale, prunes and legumes.

Vitamin K

This is a catalyst in the blood-clotting process and is essential to stop haemorrhage or miscarriage. It is found in green leafy vegetables, soya beans (non GMO), alfalfa, egg yolk, chlorophyll, oats, chestnuts, sunflower seeds and kelp.

Vitamin E

An important protection against haemorrhage and miscarriage, it also helps where there are haemorrhoids or blood clots in varicose veins and helps to normalise blood pressure. It is found in almonds, nuts, sunflower seeds, sesame oil and olive oil, brown rice, spinach and salmon.

Zinc

Zinc is used for the correct formation of brain cells and it is important that high levels are maintained throughout a pregnancy. The oral contraceptive pill depletes the liver of zinc and B Vitamins. Good sources are beef (organic, grass-fed, hormone-free) lentils, oats, oysters, shellfish, brazil nuts, pecans, pine nuts, sunflower and pumpkin seeds, and useful amounts are also found in mushrooms, spinach and soya beans (non GMO).

The above list is not exhaustive but will give you an idea of the types of foods you should be reaching for daily. It also covers the absolute essential nutrients that you must provide for you and your baby to have a healthy pregnancy.

You will see from the list that a lot of the necessary nutrients are found in green, leafy vegetables. One solution to eating enough of these to stay healthy is not just to eat plates of salad (although that is beneficial whenever possible), but instead to produce juice daily and use a plant-based protein shake to supplement your diet, which also helps keep your blood sugar levels steady. A plant-based, nutrient-rich juice, packed full of all the green leafy vegetables you require, sweetened with apple, carrot or pineapple is one of the quickest, safest and most pleasant ways to eat all that is required. It also counts towards your fluid intake each day. Into the juice, you can add wheatgrass, Spirulina, or any super- green food - all giving you a higher dose of these beneficial substances.

Guidelines on foods that are best avoided in pregnancy will list some cheeses and shellfish. They have been included in the list above as they have excellent nutritional value in the sectors covered, they appear on avoid lists because they can also carry a risk of toxicity. Alternatives are always available, so choose whatever you are comfortable with.

The mother's needs -

As mentioned before, what your baby needs is very much what you need but it is important to appreciate the changes your body will be going through. There are dozens of books that can guide you through the physical changes and reading one of these can be really informative. One I have personally loved is Well Adjusted Babies by Dr Jennifer Barham-Floreani. A large book at 700 pages, it covers every topic you could ever have a concern over.

You may not feel well at the beginning of your pregnancy, prolonged nausea and vomiting can be hard to adjust to and finding the right solution can be tricky. Hormone changes and blood-sugar levels are thought to be mostly to blame. Without synthetic hormone medication it is nearly impossible to change the new hormone levels your body is adjusting to but blood-sugar levels are much more within your control to change. Eat to make yourself healthy not to feed addictions to sugar and processed foods. Eat regularly and choose fruits, vegetables and proteins as your main dietary choices. Things with a low glycaemic index will have a more beneficial effect on your blood-sugar levels as they release their sugars into your blood stream more slowly and thus avoid the peaks and troughs that are so common with processed foods.

In most cases, this phase of nausea and even vomiting, passes within the first 12 weeks although it is possible to suffer even extreme sickness throughout the pregnancy. Do not start to hate your baby for this, however long it takes it will be over and the outcome is nothing short of magical.

Your body will change shape constantly through the months, again have faith, it knows exactly what it is doing and unhindered will carry you through the months perfectly. You can help yourself by staying fit and active, watching your posture and not allowing that increasing burden to pull you forwards and allowing you to slump. This places an incredible strain on your back which can lead to complications through delivery as your pelvis fails to move correctly through labour.

As a chiropractor who has worked in the paediatric field for decades, I consider the benefits of care for mum and baby priceless. Chiropractic care offers a 100% safe approach to wellness care through pregnancy. Every pregnant woman, in my opinion, should receive such care. Unfortunately, it is not available on the National Health Service - and probably never will be - due to the financial constraints of the overstretched system. This should not stop you seeking the support of a paediatric chiropractor for you and your baby, it will benefit you hugely.

One simple rule as your pregnancy progresses is to limit the time you sit, especially sitting slumped on sofas. This creates a backward spine-to-spine position for the baby to lie in and is one of the main contributing factors to long labours. The reason this happens is simple; the baby is responding to gravity and will move to lie at the lowest point in the uterus. For mums that sit a lot, this often means a back-to-back presentation for the baby.

If you find your baby in this position when labour starts, with each contraction the baby is turned not expelled which can lead to exhaustion before established labour even gets going. Interventions are more commonly needed to support a very tired mother. A little care through your pregnancy on postures and positions you assume regularly can go a long way to preventing this scenario.

One of the most beneficial things you can do is to talk to your baby, from the moment you are pregnant chatter away to them, sing, laugh and let them hear your voice and get to know you, keep telling them how loved and wanted they are. Talk positively and lovingly and encourage your partner to talk to the baby, too.

Most of the essential nutrients have been listed above and if you continue to live as you began in pre-pregnancy and keep your daily nutrient intake up, you should have no problems , but there are things that should be on your 'no-no' list and avoided.

1. Some processed meats carry the risk of listeriosis and so foods such as salami, pate and prosciutto should be avoided. Also in this category are foods such as shellfish and soft cheeses. As raw fish can be hazardous, sushi is best avoided.

2. Fish carries its own problems and there are three things you might like to consider when choosing to eat fish. Consider the mercury content – ask yourself what sea did the fish come from and what type of fish are you choosing? The larger fish such as swordfish and tuna bioaccummulate toxins as they live a long time and eat lots of little fish, therefore they have a high mercury content. The more toxic the sea, the worse the toxicity levels in the fish will be. Farmed fish are kept in such high numbers in such small areas, they are often packed full of antibiotics, vaccines, pesticides, fungicides and hormones in an attempt to keep them alive long enough to grow and be killed for food. Finally, consider tinned fish a no-go area. The toxin Bisphenol A is a toxic plastic chemical that lines tins and is found in just about all plastic containers. Tinned fish also contains sulphur, dioxins and sulphites, all part of the preservation process, all unnatural and all potentially harmful.

3. Avoid all trans fats. These are the most harmful fats you can eat and should be avoided throughout your life but especially when pregnant.

4. Plastic containers and drinking bottles should be avoided due to the polycarbonate chemical in the plastic. When warm this chemical leaches into the food or drink and if ever heated in the microwave will break down and spread into whatever food stuff it contacts; a point worth remembering if you are bottle- feeding your baby and heating their bottles in the microwave. These chemicals are linked to many health issues from behavioural changes to cancers.

5. Be aware of the water you drink, bottled water doesn't always represent a healthy choice. Studies have shown toxins such as pesticides, chlorine, fertilisers, hormones and solvents to be present even in natural waters fresh from the mountain spring water. The better option is to filter your own supply with a high quality alkaline filter and store it in glass bottles. This is much cheaper and healthier and one of the simpler changes you can make.

6. Avoid aspartame, this is a killer substance. It crosses the blood brain barrier and destroys brain cells, which is far from ideal for a developing baby. It is present in chewing gum, sweeteners, most processed treats and all diet drinks and food substances. Plenty of information is available on the internet about the serious health implications of consuming aspartame.

7. Best get off the tonic water, the quinine in tonic water is known to cause physical defects in embryos and the recommendation is not to consume

it while pregnant. If you are suffering with leg cramps, take more calcium and magnesium to improve the muscle function.

8. Avoid high-fructose corn syrup, this is a sweet sugar substitute that is addictive and sweeter than normal sugar but, unlike artificial sweeteners, it is a sugar. Having said that, it represents a very toxic load on your body and is best avoided. It is more common than you think and reading labels is advised. In many US formula baby milks, it is actually listed as the number one ingredient, how scary is that?

9. Minimise or eliminate caffeine, as a stimulant, it raises blood pressure and respiratory rate and places an extra strain on the kidneys trying to remove it from the body, taking some of your body's water with it and possibly adding to dehydration. Remember, caffeine is not just in coffee, it is in tea, chocolate, stimulant drinks, some medications and green tea.

10. Avoid or minimise alcohol consumption, there really is no reason why alcohol needs to be consumed while pregnant, it causes the baby damage and retards its growth processes.

11. Smoking now represents a complete taboo; nobody should ever consider smoking while pregnant. There is no excuse for inflicting such an array of addictive chemicals on your unborn child. There are about 4,000 toxic chemicals in cigarettes. Your baby could be born with addiction and suffer withdrawal as well as risking severe growth issues, retardation, miscarriage and genetic change. It is also worth considering the environments you may find yourself in while pregnant as passive smoking should also be avoided. If you give up smoking through your pregnancy but intend to smoke again once your baby is born, please bear in mind the chemicals in the cigarettes will pass to your baby through breast milk and passively in the atmosphere.

12. Avoid drugs, this seems simple on the surface but there are times when drugs are prescribed through pregnancy. Find out for yourself about the drug you are being asked to take, consider seriously why it is being suggested and consider alternatives. If you are using recreational drugs, talk to your doctor, get support and stop, you will be damaging your baby.

13. Don't be too keen to get ultrasound scans, the World Health Organisation has stated there is a distinct lack of research supporting their safety. There is no doubting they serve a purpose and it is exciting to see that first image of your baby, but it is invasive and should be viewed with caution. Have you ever wondered why all babies move and wriggle away from the probe? One theory is that it is painful for them to be hit with the ultrasonic waves. Something worth considering.

14. Source organic products for yourself and your household, cut back as far as possible on the toxic chemicals you allow into your environment. Your

skin will absorb anything you place on it and you will breathe in and touch chemicals you use around the house. Talcum powder should be avoided completely as it has been shown to have a proven link to ovarian cancer and daily use increases the risk by 41 per cent and weekly use by 36 per cent. Be careful about your skincare and make-up choices too, as your skin and lips will absorb anything you put on them. Most lipsticks contain lead and that will be directly absorbed into your system.

By following this plan you will hopefully progress through your pregnancy in a way that gives both you and your baby the best chance of staying healthy, ensuring dietary sufficiency and eliminating toxins. There are, however, other points to remember. Exercise will play a very important part in keeping you healthy, if you had time for this during the period of pre-conceptual care, you will have been able to get into the habit of regular exercise and as long as you choose an activity that is low-impact, there is no reason at all why you cannot continue with that through the months of your pregnancy. Most mum's-to-be end up with swimming and gentle walking, pregnancy yoga or pilates as their only option late in pregnancy but it is important to do all you can for as long as you can. Research proves, almost on a daily basis, the numerous health benefits of exercising regularly, so do not make the mistake of giving it up just because you're pregnant, it is most important that activity stays in your daily routine.

Sitting for prolonged periods can have a serious impact on the health of your pelvis and predisposes the baby to a posterior, back-to-back presentation. As I mentioned, this will often pre-dispose you to a longer labour than necessary and often lead to intervention to assist the delivery because labour is exhausting! Lying on your side with a support between your knees and even a small cushion under your abdomen is the best position to choose for comfort and alignment of the baby. If you are sitting at work through the day, make sure you get up and have plenty of opportunities to walk around. Ideally, you should not sit for more than 20 minutes at a time and when sitting you should ensure your knees are below your pelvis and you have a slight forward tilt on your pelvis. DO NOT sit back in your chair and lounge in it for more than just a few moments!

The last point I want to make in this section is a reminder to stay positive as your thought patterns transmit to your baby. If you are unhappy or stressed, your baby will know. Do anything you can to deal with the worries you may have and try very hard to avoid stressful situations. Talk to your baby all the time about how loved they are, how safe they are and how excited you are. You could write an affirmation that you read to them daily or just talk to them with real love and gratitude for this amazing opportunity to be their mother. This is such an important thing to do and after all the concerns about dietary choices, exercise and posture, it is the one that nearly always gets forgotten. Please do not forget it, your baby picks up on everything you think.

CHAPTER 12
The Birth and a Newborn

Whether this is your first birth or you have experienced the miracle before, one thing is sure, rarely is any woman's experience ever the same and that goes for the birth of siblings, too. My three experiences could not have been more different and my first birth plan looked like a work of fiction! Some pregnancies feel like they are destined for 10 months, not nine and at other times our little bundles arrive earlier than expected. All I can promise is that giving birth will be an experience that you will remember all your life. For you it may be a once-only event, or you may have a number of times to experience the miracle of birth. You will learn to understand yourself better than you ever have before. Within a few hours you will face fears, pain, excitement - and the unknown. You will also experience a peace and a magic that is exclusive to the experience of giving birth. To maximise the positives from this experience you should be surrounded by people you trust. People that know you well and can act in your best interests, supporting your decisions and prioritising yours and the baby's needs.

The medicalisation of the birth process has complicated what is a natural process. A process in which the body innately knows what to do. We have now been taught to trust the doctors over our bodies and instead of having a belief that the body knows what to do from the inside, procedures are forced on it from the outside. This often adds dynamics that put you on a course far removed from your intended experience.

Ideally, your baby will take about 10 hours to appear, yet so many variations occur - fast labours and slow, complicated labours pose their own problems. Interventions, pain relief and even C-section deliveries need to be carefully considered.

Our prenatal care system in the UK does not always help in the process of understanding our options and our blind trust in the medical profession often means we do not ask enough questions early on. The conveyor-belt system of antenatal check-ups means it is unusual to see the same midwife twice and so discussions about hopes and fears for the birth you want often get overlooked until you find a support network, prenatal group or family member or friend that will discuss these things with you. Your partner/husband is the obvious choice to be your rock through this process but many times their information will be as limited as yours and you will need to find someone who can educate you.

It is not uncommon to experience real panic at some of the terms and descriptions of what to expect through the birth process. Medicine makes the process clinical and takes the magic out of the moment; it treats the symptoms of labour as if they were a disease to be managed, not allowing the body to go through the perfectly-orchestrated process of birth. If you watch a wild animal or even a pet produce offspring, they are focused and calm. I watched our dog being born, I was in awe of Coco his mother, who allowed her body to grow and change while she carried on doing her doggy things and then the night her labour started she quietly took herself to a corner and moment by moment allowed her body to do what it needed to do, no panic or screaming. She allowed her instincts and the innate intelligence of her body to guide her through the process of birth. Without reading a single book or being advised to do things one way or the other, the entire process was orchestrated to perfection. I was humbled by the entire experience and so excited to see our Barney-boy born!

If you compare that to the screaming associated with a medicalised delivery, you will appreciate just how far removed we have become from our own instinctive behaviour. Everything we see and hear builds on our fear, open a magazine or turn on the television and every woman you ever see in labour is screaming. I appreciate watching a woman quietly and calmly breathe does not make great television, however, I feel there could be some middle ground here and our perception of what to expect could be made much more positive.

I am not anti-medicine for births, medical intervention has increased the survival rate of both babies and mothers and for that reason alone they should be commended and available to every expectant mother. However, from the practise of lying on your back to give birth, inductions, to elective sections for those "too posh to push" I really think we should examine our view on medicalising birth.

Currently, there is a momentum building towards home births and for many women this will represent a very positive move and exciting option. You may feel you need the security of a hospital and medical team for your baby's arrival so rest assured that will always be there. Know yourself, know where you would like to be, who you would like to assist you and how you want your birth to go. It is a very important step in keeping you relaxed and positive, allowing you to feel in control of something that has often been presented to you as a painful, terrifying process. It absolutely does not have to be that way. Keep faithfully believing in the birth you want. It took me until my third baby to actually have the birth I had always imagined. My beautiful baby girl was born at home, in a birthing pool, two weeks over her due date, I had worked with the same midwife for months and she knew me so well by the time she was coaching me through the labour she knew what I needed and when. I trusted her completely and I was so relaxed being at home. It was a very different story for my first two babies, born in hospital with every drug and intervention except a section. I recovered, my beautiful baby boys recovered but it left an emotional scar that isn't there when I reflect on my daughter's birth.

Using visualisation techniques can be extremely helpful; as athletes have proved time and time again, you can visualise your way to success. Set the intention, visualise the process in detail and run through that in your head. Combining this practise with meditation and breathing exercises can be some of the most helpful habits you get into in preparation for the arrival of your new baby. Choose music you'll listen to when you are labouring, and listen to it all the time through your pregnancy, use essential oils for calmness, plan in detail where you'll be, what you'll be wearing, who'll be around you. Add emotion to your vision and write it all down again and again in the weeks leading up to your baby's birth. These simple things are easy to do and easy not to do. Please be the person that does them, they work! Remember you are stronger than you ever imagined you could be and you and your baby will be looking at each other soon enough.

Throughout your pregnancy the topic of the birth will crop up time and time again, you may be part of a prenatal class or already part of a support group of mothers and during the months of pregnancy the discussion will repeatedly turn to the birth. This one magical day when you will get to meet your baby. What will follow will be a lifetime of unknowns, of many amazing days where you will be in awe of the life you have created. However, no other day will ever be more discussed, more strongly remembered or more longed-for than the day of your baby's birth.

There are dozens of books on the subject of pregnancy and birth and immersing yourself in these will provide you will valuable information that will enable you to cope better at all stages, this is a natural progression and you can enjoy becoming educated on the subject. Whatever choice you make, whether it's about what to eat, how to exercise, what type of birth you want or how you want to raise your child, inform yourself. Do not be led by a herd mentality, make decisions about your health and your baby's health based on sound information that you feel makes sense.

My bible for the years I was raising my children was Well Adjusted Babies by Dr Jennifer Barham-Floreani - it offers a comprehensive view of every stage of your baby's life and her chapters on birth are extremely helpful.

CHAPTER 13

Infancy

There is such a tremendous amount of thought and consideration that goes into pregnancy and birth, it can sometimes overshadow the big event – you are now a parent!! If this is your first baby, you may feel a little like a rabbit in headlights as you wonder what happens next.

A useful phrase to add to your vocabulary for the next few decades is: "it's a phase". I lived by this! It can be used as a survival mantra to anything that you are presented with over the coming years and there is deep truth in it - as almost everything is indeed a phase. It may challenge you, it may stress you, it may drive you to complete despair but just remember it is only a phase and it will pass.

Of all the challenges that you will face over the years, rarely will any seem quite as daunting as these first few weeks with your baby. You will try desperately to be the perfect mother and father and give your baby the best start. Scrabbling to understand feeding and sleeping routines, the constant cycle of changing nappies, accepting visitors, receiving helpful - and sometimes not so helpful - advice, watching your precious bundle for any sign of illness and coming to terms with the enormity of the responsibility you now have are all on your daily agenda.

There are a few simple tips that I have discovered over the years by both being a mum and working with thousands of families, they can make the difference between success and nervous breakdown!

Breast is Best

There is little arguing with the fact that there is no more perfect food for your baby than human breast milk which is designed exactly for the purpose of feeding a baby human. Anything else comes with compromise and unless you have some deep desire or reason not to feed your baby yourself, then please try, try and try again to feed your baby with breast milk. There are some wonderful help groups available that can offer practical, as well as emotional support, as you try to master this new skill. Be patient with yourself as this is can be a testing experience.

In the UK, your local NCT (National Childbirth Trust) group will have a contact to breast-feeding counsellors in your area and your health visitor should also be able to offer lots of support. If you look online for local groups and support you will realise help is out there. Ask other mothers, they very often hold the answer as to who you should be talking to.

I accept the fact that not every mother wants to breast feed, but for those that do and then find themselves unable to, there is real emotional anguish and a huge degree of fear. The instinctive feeling that their job is to feed their baby which must eat to survive, clashes with the fact they are not eating and therefore will not survive and that creates an emotional rollercoaster at a very deep primeval level.

A correctly-functioning nervous system will give your baby the best chance of latching onto the nipple and sucking correctly. Babies rely on a basic reflex called the suck reflex to perform this action; the birth process can often disrupt this and feeding will then be difficult, if not impossible. The action a baby needs to breast-feed is completely different to sucking from a bottle. They need to work their tongue hard against the roof of their mouth with a perfect seal and then they need to pump and pull the nipple to release the milk. With a bottle, they can get milk into their mouths with nothing more than a squeeze from their lips or gums.

Over the last five years, there has been a dramatic rise in the incidence of 'tongue tie', this is either the fact it was poorly diagnosed before and we now have a greater awareness of it, or there is a genuine increase with a cause yet to be identified. One theory is that the folic acid supplements given to mothers during pregnancy to prevent midline defects such as spina bifida, can cause an overgrowth of the lingual frenulum under the tongue which shortens and thickens, meaning the baby is then unable to protrude its tongue fully. The solution - once identified - is to snip the shortened tissue to release the tongue and this is usually very effective and resolves the issue completely. If you suspect this condition, please speak to your health visitor, sooner rather than later, as the difference in a baby's ability to suck once they can protrude their tongue is quite profound.

Many babies fail to thrive because of feeding issues and in my career I have found many of these issues are related to birth trauma that is correctable with pain-free adjustments by a qualified paediatric Chiropractor or Osteopath, they will be able to improve the function of your baby's nervous system and it is extremely common to see the symptoms alleviate.

When looking for a practitioner to help you and your baby, ask around within your newly- formed circle of mothers, a personal recommendation will always make you more comfortable than a cold-call to a clinic. If you fail to find a personal recommendation, then ensure you find a practitioner that deals with babies regularly. A baby is not a little adult and the same principles of care cannot be applied both to adults and babies. I recommend you find someone with extra training and specialist knowledge to assist you and your baby. The General Chiropractic Council and the General Osteopathic Council are Government-based councils that oversee these professions; they maintain the registers of qualified practitioners and can offer a useful starting point in your search.

When you are looking for clues as to the health of your baby, monitor closely their eating, sleeping, bowels actions and skin, there will always be tell-tale signs in these areas if there is strain on the nervous system.

Colic

Colic has become an overused, poorly-understood term; in its true form it represents a severe disorder of the digestive system. True colic is defined as 'three hours of violent, uncontrollable crying for at least three days a week for at least three weeks'. Babies will flail, kick, curl and go red with the strain of screaming; they appear to be in real pain that is distressing for both them and you. Colic is not necessarily associated with wind, vomiting or feeding times but is often worst in the early evening. Suggested causes vary from lactose intolerance, food allergies, constipation, structural weakness in the area of the diaphragm, reflux and finally wind issues. So many times, I have seen the impact of colic on every member of the family; the heart-breaking stress of not being able to comfort your screaming baby is real and is something no one can really understand unless they have experienced it. Tension brews within the entire family when those hours of screaming start, everyone feeling desperate and impotent as nothing seems to soothe a colicky baby. Every friend and family member has a theory on how to help and it is a hard phase to steer through. There are medications and old wives tales and most likely all will be suggested to you by someone trying to help.

The medications that are available are often no more effective than placebos and as with all drugs they carry possible side-effects that parents need to be aware of. Dietary modification, either of the mother's diet if breast-feeding, or formula choice, can have enormous benefits but it is best to follow some basic guidelines when altering your diet and understanding the reasons behind making the changes. Stress, fatigue and frustration play a huge part in worsening the effects of colic and finding a coping strategy that supports the mother-baby partnership is a very necessary step.

For breast-fed babies, it is the mother's diet that it is important to analyse. One helpful tip I give every mum is to explain that your breast milk will be approximately the meal you had eight hours before. This fact alone accounts for why so many babies struggle in the early evening. Most new mothers grab a quick breakfast usually based on dairy and wheat - most likely cereals and toast - and tea or coffee. This first meal of the day sets the tone for fluctuating blood sugar levels with peaks and troughs all day long. It places stress on insulin levels and the need for quick extra boosts to get sugar levels back up and provide the body with energy. This fuels the desire to seek out more carbohydrates and increase sugar levels fast. This is really only satisfying the mother's own energy needs and not giving the body chance for "extra" fuel to make good quality milk.

Have a think - how many times has your baby woken in the morning, had an hour or so up alert and happy then had another feed and gone back to sleep settled and content? Most days this is the pattern, even for colicky babies and it increases the frustration on the difficulties later in the day. The answer is simple, in the morning you are well rested and you are giving your baby your main meal from the night before, this is rich high-quality milk that nourishes your baby and allows for restful sleep and contentment - unlike the milk at the end of the day which is of poor quality. In addition, you are exhausted and have been feeding all day and at that point you get an unhappy, irritated baby that is unsatisfied and often in digestive pain.

The solution is to change your eating habits. The best diet and the one I suggest all new mums adopt is –

1. Eat a protein-based breakfast, not grain based. Eggs are ideal here, they are quick to prepare and have a slow energy release throughout the morning. A protein shake, if speed is needed, is a great alternative, highly nutritious and easy to eat.

2. Prepare a smoothie or fresh juice, this is packed with essential nutrients that you and your baby needs.

3. Avoid tea and coffee.

4. Avoid sugar and dairy

5. Avoid margarine and all vegetable oils.

6. Avoid artificial sweeteners, they cross the blood brain barrier and destroy both your brain cells and those of your baby.

7. Mid-morning have nuts or a snack bar or even a bowl of homemade soup. Soup is a useful thing to have constantly available, it provides nutrients and increases your fluid intake. Forget the myths about food times and food choices at each meal, if you want curry for breakfast have it!

8. Keep your water intake high, about three litres a day is correct for a breast-feeding mother. Filter your water, preferably with an alkalising filter.

9. Lunch should to be things like protein - organic meat or quinoa, salad, jacket potato (sweet if possible), soup, nuts, seeds and fresh fruit or raw vegetables.

10. Snack again mid-afternoon on nuts, homemade cakes, biscuits (they must be wheat and dairy-free) fruit or vegetables.

11. Dinner should be a repeat of anything you would choose for your lunch, not necessarily your biggest meal of the day but full of fresh ingredients.

12. All your meat should be from a source that is hormone and antibiotic-free and from grass-fed animals.

13. All your fish should come from clean seas, avoid land-farmed fish and only have large fish such as tuna and swordfish once or twice a month. These large fish bioaccumulate toxins from our polluted seas and other fish they eat.

14. Herb teas are allowed as much as you like

15. Take a high quality omega 3 supplement daily.

16. Take a high quality probiotic daily.

When making your food choices a top tip is to ask yourself "could my great-grandparents have eaten this?" and if the answer is "yes," then the chances are it is a good choice for you and the baby. But if the answer is "no," put it back and choose again!

This may all seem like an enormous effort but when you have energy, look and feel well and have a happy, contented baby you will be on top of the world. This is not a diet, it is a way of life, a way of eating that you should adopt for good health for life, and breastfeeding can kickstart your need to change. Knowing you are feeding a baby and it is your job to provide it with all the nutrients it needs to grow and develop to be strong and healthy is a fantastic feeling. It is a very important job and your baby needs you to step up and do it well. A healthy baby is the greatest gift in the world and something everyone can strive towards.

Reflux

It seems to me that the diagnosis of reflux has taken over that of colic, it is almost 'trendy' to receive this diagnosis and, in my opinion, is one of the most overused - and incorrect -terms out there. Please don't misunderstand me; true reflux is a serious issue, it requires medication until the valve at the top of the stomach closes correctly, preventing the acid in the stomach moving out of the stomach and burning the surrounding tissues. When a baby has reflux the acid from the stomach needs to be neutralised, otherwise any tissue it touches will become inflamed and damaged. Babies with true reflux, cannot lie flat, they projectile vomit, they often cough and they are very uncomfortable in any position and they most often only get some relief by being held upright. They respond very well to any medication that neutralises the acid in the stomach and will most often remain on that for up to a year - at which point almost all symptoms will be fully resolved. The closure of the valve happens during normal development, the need for medication, usually 'ranitidine' is simply to ease the symptoms through that phase and minimise the damage that could occur from the acid. It does not affect the closure of the valve in any way.

Pseudo-reflux is nothing more than a digestive irritation, through immaturity of the system, poor food choices, poor feeding habits, birth stress and many other factors, symptoms arise that make a baby irritable and uncomfortable however they are far removed from the clear symptoms of genuine reflux.

Silent Reflux is a term for reflux without the vomiting. It is often treated with the same protocol as reflux but, in my opinion, there are many other more helpful approaches to try with babies in this category. Chiropractic or osteopathic treatments can be very beneficial, dietary changes, adopting different positional habits, addressing any feeding issues and assessing the baby for other areas of concern may give a fuller picture as to where problems lie.

Bottle-fed babies

Many mothers choose not to breast-feed and many more may try, encounter problems and through lack of support, upset and frustration often very reluctantly and sadly, give up. The options are then limited to formula milks or prescription hydrolysed milks for babies with cow's milk allergies. Formula milks are produced for the mass market and all contain very similar ingredients, however, they do vary and I have seen many babies with a preference both on health and taste grounds. It is always worth trying different milks if your baby is struggling on one. All formula milks are based on cow's milk. They contain large proteins and lactose, which is the sugar in milk. They are most commonly sweetened with high fructose corn syrup and supplemented with synthetic vitamins and minerals. They offer a growing baby calories, nutrients and fluid and unless there is a serious intolerance to the milk the baby will grow. It is not uncommon to hear of food intolerances and allergies to formula milks as the large proteins in the milk pass through the holes in an infant's bowel wall directly into their bloodstream, setting up an immune response. The holes in the baby's bowel lining are there for a reason, described as a leaky gut they are there to allow antibodies from a mother's breast milk to pass into the blood stream and protect the baby while it builds the strength of its own immune system. These antibodies are large and, without the holes, they would not be able to get into the baby's system. Unfortunately, those same holes allow the passage of the large dairy proteins into the bloodstream and induce an immune crisis - either immediately or sometimes many years later.

Talking poo!

Our bowel actions give us key clues as to the true state of our digestive system and this stays true for our entire lives. However, as a new mother you can glean a lot of information about the health of your baby from the frequency, colour and consistency of what ends up in your baby's nappies.

Changes of any type are significant and are best not ignored. Some are quickly explainable and also short-lived, while others are the warning signs of a change in the function of the digestive system.

Breast-fed babies can go up to three weeks without a bowel action; they are content, comfortable, have good weight gain and show no signs of other health issues, yet could very easily be labelled constipated. What is happening is that the baby is using every bit of the milk that is being delivered to it. As long as there is good steady weight gain, there is absolutely nothing to worry about. This scenario occurs most commonly when the mother has a "perfect" diet as there are no toxins, no waste and therefore no poo! However, if this is your baby please be mindful that it is still important to have lots of wet nappies and a content baby.

More commonly, a baby will have frequent, soft, pain-free bowel actions up to six times a day, often described as looking like a korma curry with seeds in! This is another perfectly normal situation and as long as there is good weight gain and feeding is not excessive, this would be classed as normal and healthy. As with most health issues, it is change that should alert us to something not being right. Keeping a close eye on your baby's bowel motions and asking yourself what could be the cause if you see changes is a smart and diligent approach. Because the constituents of formula milk are different to breast milk, you will see a different type of poo from bottle-fed babies. Their waste matter is made up of different food types and you can expect anything from korma-type yellow, soft, seedy stools, to better-formed, darker-coloured, less frequent bowel actions. This in itself can cause a baby more issues as they are harder to process and pass for a very immature system.

Babies can develop acute bouts of diarrhoea. If this happens to your baby your primary concern should be dehydration. Whatever the cause, bacteria, virus, food or side effects of drugs, always keep a very close eye on a sick baby and ensure they are well hydrated at all times. If severe dehydration becomes an issue, they will become very lethargic, often floppy and non-responsive, you may notice the fontanelle (soft spot on their heads) becomes concave and in these cases they must go to hospital quickly to be placed on a drip to rehydrate them. I always teach parents that if your baby is screaming and making noise you have less to worry about than if they go very quiet, lethargic and floppy.

If you are unlucky enough to have a baby that gets full-blown gastroenteritis, after the illness watch that they do not develop a sensitivity to the sugar in milk, this is quite a common occurrence. It appears that the milk sugar, lactose, causes a real irritation to many babies and this will be seen as frequent, frothy, very smelly bowel actions. The only way to help your baby is to use a lactose-free formula/milk for a period of time and support the healing of the bowel with a baby powder probiotic available from good quality, independent health food shops or online.

Vaccinations

Is there a more controversial topic? Even though I know this is a really emotive topic, I knew this book would not be complete without it.

Whatever your viewpoint is, no parent enters lightly into the vaccination programme of their child. Vaccinating for personal safety or herd immunity or abstaining completely, all come with tough decisions. Sometime, even getting two parents to agree is the toughest of all. Tensions brew in families where parents have opposing views, each with equally strong beliefs about vaccinations. There are pros and cons and all parties can put compelling arguments forward that leave you as parents confused and scared. Without wanting to compound your confusion, there are some facts worth noting.

All vaccines, based on either dead or attenuated agents (antigens) are designed to enter the body and stimulate the immune system into action. Presenting the body with an exposure to a weakened form of possibly a deadly disease and allowing it to recognise and build antibodies to that, seems on the surface, a safe and sensible thing to do. However, the process of vaccinating in most cases puts the substance directly into the bloodstream, which is a very different route than would occur naturally and completely bypasses the body's locally-based immune response which is in something called the gut-associated lymph tissue which is responsible for 75% of our ability to fight off diseases.

The use of multiple vaccines is now common practise, a situation that would never occur in nature. Have a think.....when in nature are people exposed to measles, mumps and rubella or diphtheria, polio and tetanus in the same day? There has been endless controversy over the MMR vaccine and its links to autism and this triple vaccine does seem to have the potential to wreak havoc in the body. You may be of the view there is no smoke without fire and even if there has not been evidential proof of the link, you only need to see a child or speak to a parent of an affected child to see that there are some cases where, for whatever reason, appear to have a clear link between the administration of a vaccine and a severe and irreversible change in the health of that child.

A child can receive up to 14 vaccinations in their first three years of life. This includes at least 32 exposures to 12 different infectious diseases. Most vaccines are given as combinations and many boosters are given throughout the first three years.

Vaccines historically contained thimerosal, a derivative of mercury, used as a preservative for the vaccine. For decades, this toxic, heavy metal was injected almost directly into the bloodstream of babies together with the vaccine. Nowadays, vaccines have had the thimerosal removed and it has been replaced by aluminium. Knowing which vaccinations are being given when and asking questions before your baby is vaccinated is a smart move. I suggest you even ask to keep the packaging from the vaccines so you are 100% sure of the ingredients and side-effects of your baby's vaccine, this can be a powerful safeguard should the absolute worst happen and your baby or child has a reaction.

Number one rule when your baby is being vaccinated is to ensure they are completely well prior to the vaccine. To me, that means they are happy, content, symptom free in all areas, have no cough, no runny nose, no skin disorders, no digestive upsets, colic, wind or reflux, no constipation, no diarrhoea or sleep issues. Vaccines place an incredible strain on a very young immature system and you will be more confident that your baby is strong and healthy and able to cope well if you know they were really well before the vaccines. There is an intrinsic link between the nervous system and the immune system so if your baby has been under paediatric chiropractic or osteopathic care from birth, this will help ensure that their nervous system is functioning at an optimal level.

After vaccinations, do not be surprised if your baby is unwell - an increase in temperature and lethargy are completely normal signs. The body will always raise its temperature when it finds itself under invasion and you do it no favours by artificially lowering it with medication. In fact, you make it much harder for the body to respond to the vaccination. It is a short term gain of comfort for a long term loss of immunity. Going right back to basics, you'll remember me saying that the body always has an appropriate response to any particular circumstance and it is always the best response possible. Our bodies have our best interest at heart! Producing a fever is what our bodies are programmed to do when we have a foreign invader in us. It is the quickest and smartest way to get well again. It takes approximately four days to build antibodies to an infection and in that period of time the body is defenceless except for its ability to raise the body temperature. Because bacteria and viruses cannot survive at higher than normal body temperatures, if the body is given time and allowed to raise the temperature, the impact of the vaccine will be less and the reaction from the immune system strong and appropriate. Understanding the theory of this and living it in practise are two very different things. It is very hard to see your baby unwell knowing there is a quick fix in a dose of medication. All I can do is encourage you to have a long-term view and have lots of cuddle time. Keep fluid levels up and watch your baby/child very carefully, keep them calm and quiet for a few days after a vaccine. After four days, your baby's immune system will start to produce the exact antibodies it needs to build a long-term defence against that particular disease and, at that point, the entire system is calmer and your baby will seem well again.

As I mentioned before, it is often hard to get independent advice on the subject of vaccinations as there seem to be two diametrically opposed camps and that is enough to confuse anyone. The doctors and drug companies make money out of vaccination programmes and all their research is designed to support the benefit of vaccination.

The other camp is about exposing what they see in this corrupt system and highlighting the dangers to your baby of such strong vaccination programmes. Faced with all this pressure it is very hard to know how to do the right thing.

My best advice is to read and research for yourself. Then as a couple you should try and find a way in which you are both comfortable with your decision as you must be prepared to live with the consequences of a worst case scenario in either decision. If you can settle yourselves to that, you will be fine with your choice. For example you may feel you could never live with yourself if you injected your baby and they got autism or worse, you decide you would rather take your chances with nature. Or you may feel that you could never live with yourself if you did not vaccinate and your baby caught a killer disease. I completely appreciate the intensity of this decision for any parents, it really is a lose, lose situation because the worst case outcome from either decision is horrific.

Nobody said being a parent would be easy!

Two excellent books on this topic are "What Doctors May Not Tell you about Children's Vaccinations" by Stephanie Cave and Well Adjusted Babies" by Jennifer Barham-Floreani.

....

What Doctors May Not Tell You about Children's Vaccination is a book which has the potential to be very alternative but I was impressed with its ability to educate and steer parents through the vaccination minefield. It will give you information on what to watch out for and how to request particular vaccines at particular times. It is not completely unbiased (no book ever is!) but it is a good read.

We are lucky in the UK because, unlike the USA, vaccination programmes are not yet compulsory. We still have the freedom of choice and no school place will be denied if your child is not vaccinated. It would be a travesty if that situation were ever to change and the choice for your child's wellbeing was taken out of your hands. Let's pray that day never arrives.

Sleep

Apart from feeding issues this is a hot topic! We all dream of the perfect baby that enters our life and does not disrupt it completely, this is never more true than our desire to still have a full night's sleep after our newborn arrives. I hate to be the bringer of bad news but this is not going to happen for many weeks. Your newborn baby may be an absolute angel but they still need regular food and that means disturbed nights. On the plus side, those hours spent with your baby in the quiet of the night can be some of the most magical bonding moments you will ever have.

Breast or bottle fed, demand or routine, your nights will be an extension of the day's feeding pattern. Breast-fed babies often feed more regularly as the milk is easier to digest and therefore passes through the digestive system more quickly than formula feeds. Many parents utilise that fact to try and get their babies to sleep longer by filling them with formula feed at bedtime, or offering a dream feed. As discussed in the feeding section, there are pros and cons to either feeding choice but understanding how feeding choices can affect sleep patterns I think you may find very useful.

A baby should have periods of deep sleep and contented wakeful times. They work on a 24-hour cycle, initially not differentiating night from day until they are a few weeks old. After a few weeks, they can settle into longer periods of sleep through the night and longer periods awake through the day. This is led by hormone changes in the brain and daylight patterns, even small babies benefit from darkness to trigger sleep. Routine is incredibly important, having a wind-down period to precede bedtime is a great routine to establish even at a very young age.

There are numerous sleeping options to consider and all are acceptable in the first few weeks, co-sleeping, crib by the bed, cot with a baby monitor, shared rooms, single rooms, the options are endless. However, as the months tick by, you may find yourself wanting to progress to a different option. You may have been co-sleeping with your newborn but never intended to keep it up. All babies would prefer to be close to you ALL the time, it helps them feel safe and they are reluctant to break that bond. As they get older they will get smarter and smarter at manipulating you to get exactly what they want. If you want to continue to co-sleep with your baby that is absolutely fine and for some parents co-sleeping is an important part of parenting and something they enjoy for many years. For other parents, they find it is something that they started and then find hard to break the habit. My best advice is to stay strong, work together as parents to find the best solution for breaking that habit that suits your family situation. Phasing change or going "cold turkey" I've heard success and failure stories from them all and I would suggest that you do what is right for you as a family. There are endless books written on this topic and so much more online, if this is the stage you are struggling with then read up about it and talk to other parents someone will have tried something that will work for you, too. It will seem like the blink of an eye until you have a teenager that you can't stop sleeping! It's all a phase and this sleep deprivation phase - although extremely hard - will pass, I promise!

There are a few sleep issues to be aware of; firstly a baby that sleeps all the time, especially if it falls asleep early in a feed and needs to be constantly woken to finish the feed. This most often occurs in the first few weeks of life and could be an alarm sign for a baby that has been traumatised by the birth process. Many births present physical trauma to the baby, remember they are on the inside of all those contractions! They often have physical bruises and swelling as well as misshapen heads because of high pressure and interventions.

The excess sleeping is equivalent to a semi-coma and a clear sign that your baby is struggling to be conscious. Repair the damage from the birth process with some corrective chiropractic or osteopathic care and feeding and sleeping will almost certainly improve. Think of it as a traumatised baby will even sacrifice feeding for sleep in an attempt to heal themselves and this often presents as babies that fail to thrive and have very slow weight gain. Sadly, I find this is often blamed on breast-feeding and mothers are encouraged to move their babies onto a bottle in an attempt to help their baby gain more weight. This approach usually helps the weight gain but does nothing to address the underlying issue of the excessive sleeping and irritation into the nervous system.

This sleepy phase usually only lasts a few weeks and then the baby becomes more alert again. A huge advantage can be gained by seeking help early on and getting your baby to a paediatric cranial osteopath or chiropractor. Their treatment will normalise nervous system function and should speed up the healing process. Long, traumatic labours are particularly significant in the history of these babies.

A baby that won't sleep – that dreaded scenario! Remember babies should sleep; if you have a baby that will not sleep there is usually something wrong. They can be reacting to foods, illness, birth trauma or the environment but whatever the cause it should be addressed for the sanity of the whole family! Again, my best advice is to get your baby checked as soon as possible after birth. Things to look out for are babies that are rigid, appear to have excellent head control (far too good for their age) and usually dislike sitting, they startle very easily and often dislike being held and restrained.

Sleep position – another highly controversial topic is the "back-to-sleep" campaign, founded in 1994, it has pushed hard to get babies sleeping on their backs. This has led to a rise in the incidence of flat spots on babies' heads as constant external pressure is applied to the cranial bones. This condition called plagiocephaly is not caused by the sleep position but it is aggravated by it, hence it is being seen more frequently since the majority of babies have been placed on their backs at night. Proactive Chiropractic or Osteopathic care is very important as the window for changing these flatspots is only the first 12 months, this is the time frame where head growth is the fastest and offers the greatest opportunity for resolution.

For generations, babies have slept on their tummies and these flat spots were not seen in these high numbers. Tummy sleeping is helpful for digestive issues and brain development so if you are comfortable with the idea then your baby will be happy in that position.

Weaning

One of the most discussed and worried over phases in a baby's development - what to introduce and when? An entire industry has grown up around baby food, first foods, follow-on foods, recipes for babies, recipes for toddlers the list is endless and behind every one, there is someone trying to make money. Do they have the health of your baby as their priority; I think it would be naïve to answer yes to that. Do they want to harm your baby? Absolutely not but they do want to make a profit and they will market hard to you to ensure they do. How did we ever know what to feed a baby before television or the internet?

When should you wean your baby?

Your answer to this will depend very much on your age, the current directives and your past experience if you have other children. It is often a phase that can be rushed into, especially if there have been any feeding or sleep issues in those early months. The thought of sleep again because a baby is put down with a full tummy seems like such a simple solution, but it can compound an already stressed system and create even more issues. If you are weaning your baby because it suits you, rather than them, this is usually the moment that you encounter problems. Stressed young systems can hit overload and more symptoms will appear. For example, you can take an irritable baby that does not sleep well and maybe has a little eczema and after introducing solids you have an irritable baby with eczema and now constipation too, this often happens if you wean too soon on the wrong foods.

A better approach may be to wait until you have a settled baby, one that is hitting their milestones well, that had developed some routine to eating and sleeping, that has a robust immune system and a very predictable digestive system. If you are unsure, try using the tried and tested method of waiting for your baby to cut at least four teeth before you consider weaning. This is my preferred method as I feel it is nature's way of saying "ok I'm ready to chew now" it also indicates that the stomach acid is getting stronger and will be better able to digest what is sent down. The rising signs of acidity can often be seen around the mouth as redness and as bouts of nappy rash. This is due to the increased acidity of the saliva and urine. It settles each time a tooth cuts.

If you have the restraint to wait until your baby is ready for food and work with them, not against them, you will usually have a much smoother transition. Be gentle on your baby's system and I suggest you start with pureed organic fruit and vegetables, these are packed with amazing nutrients and easy to digest than baby rice which is mass-produced, highly-processed, nutrient-void grain.

Weaning recommendations have changed so much over the last 30 years. First it was three months, then six months then four months and has now settled around six months. Following the advice for a minimum age is helpful for some parents but allow your baby to tell you, look for other signs, especially the cutting of teeth. If you introduce solid food thinking your baby will sleep and become settled once they are on it, you may have a shock when that doesn't happen.

Beginning with organic fruit and vegetables; cooked and pureed means you will know exactly what is in it. Freeze what you make in an ice tray and bring out small portions each day. Milk should still be your baby's main source of food as you transition them onto solids.

The progression onto more and more solid food can be done at your pace; there are so many recipes and so much information out there. Your main concern should be the starting point, do not be too keen, it is very hard to go back and undo the introduction of solid food!

Some babies are naturals at eating solid food whilst others struggle with the swallowing action, the chewing action and even the texture. Some are very reluctant to have anything other than breast or bottle as a way to get fed. Some are clean eaters and others are best fed in a bath! Remember it is a phase, it will pass, they will master it. Let food be interesting and enjoyable and cook from scratch using organic foods. Many parents enjoy baby-led weaning, meaning you allow your baby to feed themselves, they choose their food off the plate and eat without assistance, again this can be very messy, prepare for it! If there are siblings in the house they can be both a help or a hindrance, if they are fussy eaters, the chances are your baby will develop those traits, if they enjoy their food they will tend to be a positive role model for that behaviour. Keep foods colourful and textures varied. There are lots of cheat ways to get healthy foods into children, try and remember you are the boss. Their growth and health is dependent on you making smart food choices for them. Watch out for foods that make them irritable or ill, flare skin issues, a change in bowel actions, make them mucussy or create challenging behaviours. These are best removed.

Sugar is the most common food that children have a problem with as they become driven by an addiction to it. When you start weaning, if you keep sugars to a minimum and expose your baby to many colours, textures and flavours, they will not be drawn only to sugar and this will make your job very much easier as they grow. Try and include healthy fats in your baby's diet from an early stage. Avocados offer the best source of these and represent a perfect whole food for your baby. They are packed with essential omega fats and can be eaten daily as a food for your baby.

Processed grains are always best avoided; there is never a good time to give a child cereals, white bread, white pasta, pastries or biscuits. All those grains turn to glue in the digestive system and they are best cut out or never introduced.

Whole grains such as organic brown rice, quinoa, millet, amaranth and spelt are best introduced after 12 months in small amounts and not more than once a day.

Most meals should consist of fruits and vegetables, pureed in those early weeks, with the introduction of some organic grass-fed meats after four months or more of solid food intake.

If you can, keep a close eye on bowel actions and the condition of the skin throughout this transitional phase, they will give you a quick indicator that things are doing well internally, or in some cases, not so well.

If you have been diligent with breast-feeding and keeping dairy out of your diet to avoid any reaction by your baby, you may be wondering what to do as you wean. Obviously, you can keep breast-feeding going for as long as it works for you and your baby but this tends to become less frequent as your baby gets nutrients from other sources, when the time comes to stop all together a good alternative for small drinks and for cooking with are plant, oat or nut-based milks. Water is always preferred by children and it is easy to maintain that preference as long as sweet juices are not offered. It is best to avoid soya as it is allergenic, acidic, a GMO crop and contains phyto-oestrogens, once hailed as having health-giving properties it is now regarded as a concern, especially to boys.

If you personally have had no issues with dairy protein digestion and your baby appears to have coped well with formula feeds, then you may still like to consider making a swap to plant-based milks as they offer a great alternative and have an alkalising effect on the body. Human beings lose the enzymes to break down milk-based proteins from about three years of age, so once those enzymes are gone, the milk presents quite a problem to our digestive system when it needs to be broken down. It is a smart decision to take that added stress away and use a product that is easier to digest.

Calcium, as discussed in detail in an earlier chapter, is found in higher quantities and in a more absorbable form when ingested as green, leafy vegetables. Adding spinach to sauces and purees is an amazing way to provide your baby with high levels of calcium.

This is far from all the issues you may encounter in these early years but after decades raising three children and working with babies these are the most common and the simplest solutions I have found. They have worked for so many parents that I wanted to share them all with you. Much of what I have learnt has not come easily - two years of no sleep with my first baby, severe eczema on my daughter and feeding issues and digestive upsets seemed to be the norm for many years. Finding a way through it and then passing on what I have learnt has enabled me to make many parents' journeys much smoother than mine.

I have a deep belief that there is nothing stronger than a mother's instinct, you will never find me fobbing off a single concern from any parent. If you feel things aren't right, that's good enough for me, something isn't right.

If in your gut you feel something isn't the way it should be, please be proactive in solving the issue because once it's solved you will have the parenting experience you dreamt of.

I always say: "happy baby equals a happy family!"

CHAPTER 14

Toddlers!

By three years old, your toddler should be able to eat everything on the healthy eating list. It is around this age that they are can cope with nuts, raw carrots and popcorn without the risk of choking. Shellfish can be introduced with a reduced fear of developing a susceptibility to allergy. Caution is needed about shellfish, as with all meats and fish knowing the source of the product is extremely important. Most shellfish are bottom- feeders and as such can accumulate all sorts of toxins if those are present in the water.

In an ideal world this is the first age at which a child should have had any exposure to white sugar. This is a toxic, highly-processed substance devoid of all nutrients and offering only calorie content and due to its highly-addictive traits, it is a good one to steer clear of for as long as you possibly can.

One very significant event happens at around three years old; when the enzymes required to breakdown milk proteins are lost. The significance of this event is often overlooked, both by children and adults, as dairy products continue to be in our diets long after weaning. The enzyme is lost for no other reason than nature would expect us to be weaned by three years old and therefore the necessity to continue to produce the enzymes required for the breakdown of the product should no longer be required. We have, however, ignored nature by continuing to keep dairy proteins in our diets.

Just to emphasise this very important fact - anyone aged three or older does not possess the ability to breakdown dairy proteins by use of a specific enzyme. Some will get digested by stomach acids and other enzyme activity but the system will not be as intended and there are often health consequences seen in the form of allergies that develop with prolonged ingestion of this food.

Skin

Skin is classed as an organ system in the body. It is the largest organ in our bodies and yet we probably never think of it in any other way than a barrier to the outside world. However, it is a moving, constantly renewing organ that protects us from external injury, entry of bacteria and viruses, radiation and chemicals; it regulates our temperature with its ability to respond to hot or cold; it detoxifies our system via our sweat glands; it allows us to sense via an intricate system of nerve endings capable of relaying messages to our brain detecting all sensations from light touch to pain and it is key in our production of Vitamin D.

In newborn babies, their body systems are not fully developed, they will spend many years growing and developing full function and the skin organ is no different. A baby will not control temperature well through sweating or shivering, it will not have good chemical, radiation, bacterial or viral protection and it will not sense with the same sensitivity as our adult skin does. These functions will develop and become fine-tuned over years. However, the skin performs one function very well even from being very young, it is an excellent exit route for toxic substances within the body. With this in mind, the signs to watch for are dry, red, cracked, irritated areas of skin. It is important that this is attended to immediately; think what might have been applied to the skin and what could possibly have caused the reaction. Pure is definitely best in the case of children's skin, keeping all chemical toxins to a minimum is the least that is required if you want to avoid skin reactions. Choose organic baby products, vegan products and ones that have a food standard rating. If you would not put it in your mouth, why would you put it on your skin? Be wary of some of our tap water as it can be acidic and harsh on sensitive skin.

Sun protection is an important consideration for most parents. It is extremely important not to let your baby get burnt, yet when they start running around and wanting to be outdoors more and more it can become a challenge to protect their skin. Burnt skin signifies damaged skin and can lead to scarring or permanently changed cells. However, it is also extremely important to allow your child's skin to be exposed to the sun so they can make enough vitamin D to grow healthy bones. Our English climate, inside living and obsession with sunscreens is currently producing a rise in the incidence of rickets (a childhood disease involving weak bones and indicative of Vitamin D deficiency). It is a sad reflection that such a disease is resurfacing in the modern world where deficiencies should be a thing of the past. This resurgence of rickets has resulted from a fear of skin cancer from sun exposure and has neglected to appreciate the health benefits that a safe exposure to sun can give us.

Avoiding the midday sun while still allowing skin exposure to the sun during the less intense morning and late afternoon times is a safe way to get sunlight on the skin. Twenty to 30 minutes a day of sunlight on our skin will boost Vitamin D production and is safe and healthy. Our arms, legs and face need to be exposed to have 40 per cent of our body's skin able to absorb sunlight. If you are out in the midday sun, an organic mineral sun screen should be applied to skin that is exposed and light clothing worn. In the UK, our sun is too low in the sky and of too low an intensity to stimulate the body to make Vitamin D in the winter months and it is a good idea to take a Vitamin D supplement for six months of the year. Children's spray Vitamin D is readily available now and an easy way to ensure they are getting the supplement that they need October to April.

Skin also acts as an exit route for internal toxins and as such is a great indicator of problems that may be brewing internally. Toxins that cause skin eruptions will almost exclusively have to have been ingested which means they are either in the food we eat or medications we may be taking. With babies, their food supply is very limited and should be scrutinised if any skin irritation is present. With toddlers, this becomes a little more complicated! Food diaries can be really useful, if you can write down everything that is eaten or drunk for seven days you will see patterns appearing and you will then be able to remove things you feel are culprits and watch for the skin to improve. You can always then do a challenge test by reintroducing something you feel is irritating and watch what happens to the skin. It is a fast response so you should get answers very quickly. You can do this under guidance or just by yourself, it's simple enough to do, the food diary is the secret to knowing where to start.

Poo!

Just like the skin, the digestive system is also an exit route for waste material and what cannot be used will be eliminated. In babies, this is easy as dozens of nappy changes take you to the exit end and you can quickly and easily make an assessment on colour, consistency and frequency. Remember, that change is significant so do not ignore it, monitor it and think what you might have altered in the 12 hours prior to the changes. Has there been some new food introduced, less feeds, any medications or are there any other signs of illness?

If the bowel actions of a toddler or child change, the same rules apply, look for other signs of illness but also look at their food intake. Our digestion is an easy in and out system -remember, if we put rubbish in we will more than likely get a rubbish result at the other end!

Normal bowel actions for a toddler on solid food should be two or three times a day, cause them no pain and be brown in colour, soft but formed and not be too offensive smelling.

It is a transitional age as far as nappies are concerned, some toddlers are fast to potty train and gain both bladder and bowel control, while others are much slower. Try to work with your child and not give them too much fear around these elimination actions!

Children that get fearful often cause themselves terrible constipation issues by hanging on and just refusing to have a poo. It is not uncommon for laxatives to be given to small children and yet there is so much that can be done with hydration and diet that would negate the need for medication.

A child's psychological state has an impact on their bowel activity so it's always a good idea to consider if there is stress in the household or around them as they can react with digestive symptoms.

Toddlers are very prone to diarrhoea and as long as this is short-lived, there are rarely any ongoing issues, a full-blown gastroenteritis can cause long-term problems especially with the breakdown of milk sugars. This is not a problem if your child is dairy-free but if they eat dairy, they very often get a post-infection reaction. The solution is to eliminate the cause for a period of time, take dairy away, and give a probiotic to repair and rebalance the bowel microbes.

Milestones

My eldest walked at nine months, my middle child shuffled around on his bottom, never crawling and my daughter must have read a text book on development and did it to the letter - taking her first steps on her first birthday! They are all different. Watching your child hit milestones can put undue pressure on parents, and peer pressure mounts as friends' children achieve goals first. Looking at milestones does serve a purpose and gives a baseline to work from by monitoring levels reached, achieved and mastered. The absence of a stage is significant and something that rings alarm bells in paediatric circles. When my son didn't crawl I knew we had to be proactive and ensure that neurologically the development was still there. I see in practice often the thrill on parents' faces as their baby is going straight to stand and walk and is missing out crawling. It is not that walking at ten months is not a phenomenal feat for the brain to coordinate and master, it is the fact that the child missed out crawling that may be significant and the obvious question that should be asked and answered is why?

Why would the brain miss out a phase it is programmed to pass through? An adaptive event must occur within its internal wiring for that to happen. So milestones are not to be smugly talked about as parents meet as much as they are to be noted for order of achievement.

If you have a child you are concerned about it, is always better to be proactive rather than reactive. It is not a time to bury your head in the sand, it is time to make yourself heard, get your child assessed and find out what is wrong. Little often quite cute, quirky habits can be early tell tale signs that things are not quite developing in the correct order. Help is at hand both with chiropractic care and medical screenings and your parental instincts are key here, if you feel something is wrong, voice it!

The Terrible Twos!

Who said they had to be terrible? They don't have to be that way, we have all witnessed some appalling tantrums from friends' children and strangers. Moments where you would just like to slunk away or have the ground swallow you up as this little tot has found a way to completely control you. We have also seen some beautifully behaved children so know they do exist! Your approach is best when multifaceted. If you have a child that is receiving all its innate requirements for good health and wellbeing, how can you have an emotional breakdown? Tantrums are either led by addiction for a food substance, in which case they appear no less serious than a heroin addict being denied their next fix; or by an emotional need that requires filling.

If you have a child whose body wants sugar you will know about it and so will the rest of the supermarket! This is actually one of the simplest issues to address as the physical addiction can be cleared out of the body in 48 hours with the correct advice and support. After that time, the addiction is emotional not chemical. So if you have a child that holds you hostage at the sweet counter then you might like to try the following advice.

What to do when your child is addicted to sugar

There is no simple way around this, you just have to remove all the sugar from the diet and anything the body can turn into sugar. This is not a pleasant phase! This is an ugly, "I'm an addict" sort of phase. It is the phase where you have to be united and strong and not give in to demands, tantrums or any other strategy that might be played out and these can be many. It lasts about 48 to 72 hours and should be planned for in detail. If you can talk to your child and make them understand that there are going to be some food changes then do so but if not, just go for it! Possibly the whole family could go through the change of diet as it is really good that all our bodies can to get a rest from high sugar intake.

Behind the change is the idea that the bowel flora must be allowed to resume new levels. The bacteria and fungus that live off sugar must die off and the other less strong but vital ones must be encouraged back to full numbers. This takes time but the initial phase is quick. Our bowel microbes renew every three days.

- You will need a child probiotic (the highest quality you can buy) which is usually in powder form for young children and can be added to any fluid or food.

- You will need exercise and day activities designed around keeping your child really happy, well exercised and preferably outdoors.

- You will need to choose foods with a very low glycemic index – 50 or below. No wheat, fruit juice, fresh fruit, squash, biscuits, sweets, sweet yoghurts, pastry, ice-cream, chocolate, cakes or yeast-based products should be consumed.

In their place, your child will need a diet based around fresh vegetables, meat, potatoes, preferably sweet potatoes, nuts, seeds, pulses, water, fresh vegetable juice with a little apple or pineapple for taste (but only if made in a juicer and drunk immediately) eggs, milk (best options are organic rice milk, coconut, almond, oat or sesame milk)

The emotional link to sugar can be harder to break than the physical one. There is often a connection with sugar being given as a reward, "if you're good for mummy I'll buy you some sweeties afterwards" – sound familiar?? Bribery is something that every non-parent swears they will never use and every parent succumbs to once they realise what a fantastic tool it is to get what you need, whether that is peace and quiet or good behaviour, in the end everyone succumbs! There are many healthy ways to reward a child and sugar-based treats do not have to be one of them. You will probably end up with some weird and wonderful collections of things over the years and have some great trips out all based around the promise of a reward. Whenever you doubt this approach, listen to the little voice in your head saying why reward with something that is harmful, why give the child you adore something that will make them less well just because it is easier and they want it? Small children want quality time and love and that is their greatest reward.

A word of caution, there is a very strong link between boredom and eating, children that are not stimulated will eat without limit. So if you have a child in front of the television they will munch away and never really feel full. In this scenario you have two options, use this mindless hand-to-mouth action to get healthy foods into your child or stop the TV time and get your children active. A combination of both will be most advantageous to your child.

There is a saying about white foods being the white man's death; it goes from white sugar, white flour, white rice, white milk, man in white coat treating with white pills, white man's diseases and ends in white man's early death.

Of all the foods white sugar and processed white foods are the worst you will ever give your child, so if you are reading this and learning about health while your children are still young enough, or maybe not even born yet then please just never introduce them, or in minimal amounts so not to be obsessive and if you are learning this information when your child is older and has already developed a taste/addiction to them you will have to change their diet to remove the culprit foods and educate your child to better choices. You should make these changes as a family, never isolate a child and continue to do wrong yourself, they will view that as unfair and confusing and they would be right!

School years

From 4 to 18 years, children enter a system of education that is disciplined and regimented and intended to guide an average child through learning basic skills in all areas of development from social to intellectual. This happens outside the family environment and can be quite traumatic for some children as they have to learn new rules and conform to systems they are not used to. The entire process of education is staged, monitored and regulated with the aim to get the majority of children from point A to point B and equipped to enter the wider world. The key words here are average and majority and not all children fit this band. More and more children have their own personal difficulties and health issues and these are often seen most markedly when they are in a class of other children of the same age. Weight issues, height differences, stamina, co-ordination, speech, reading, writing and social interaction are all observed very differently when comparisons are made in a peer group.

It is sometimes easy to ignore developmental issues in a child as they exist at home in isolation and difficulties are often catered for or put down as quirky. This can be a dangerous road to take as it can often result in action not been taken to help a child get over their issues.

One of the main problems that arise in children under ten are co-ordination issues and learning problems at school. These usually surface about five to seven years old when a teacher flags up some concerns, or as a parent you realise that your child is not growing out of a problem. There are currently a lot of "labels" out there and many parents have to go through endless assessments to get one of these "labels" to ensure extra support and help for their child. This can be detrimental on many levels but in most cases unavoidable due the protocols we have in place within the health and education systems.

I think sometimes we forget the basics and from what I have witnessed over the years profound improvement can be seen in children when you support good posture, ensure healthy nutrition, get your child enjoying exercise and use chiropractic care to improve the function of their nervous system.

Here is a useful phrase that i teach all the parents I see, "do not ignore the niggles" if you have a child that complains about something - listen; if you see something that doesn't look right – instigate some investigation; if you just get a gut feeling - trust it, you are the parents, you know this human being better than any other person on the planet and they need you to be watching out for them as they grow up. So if you spot that your child rolls their feet in, waddles like a duck, runs awkwardly, has poor co-ordination, struggles with any aspect of school work, has poor concentration, poor sleep, weight issues, general health issues or even a confirmed diagnosis of illness get them checked, do not ignore the symptom. Assist them to grow out of their problem not into it.

A Complete Lifestyle Diet for Children

Without wanting to sound too repetitive the rules that we should help our children live by are simple - supply the body with all the nutrients it requires for growth, repair and energy and limit toxic substances in their diet.

My 5 top tips for children daily

Drink at least 1 litre of fresh water a day - (use the weight in pounds divided by two equation to work out how many fluid ounces your child should drink each day)

Eat fresh, raw organic fruits and vegetables everyday - at least five portions

Take omega 3 oils daily

Avoid processed white foods of all descriptions

Avoid artificial sweeteners

On the exercise front, get at least 30 minutes of heart pounding exercise each day. For children this needs to be in game form as it has to be fun to get them to do it! Kids are smart, they love fun!

Limit TV time to one hour a day between 2 and 10 years old.

Make sure your child goes to bed at a suitable time; they require ten to 12 hours a night in this age group. Keep a strict bedtime routine that includes a wind-down and no TV before bed and no computer or electronic games. Ensuring these are all kept out of the bedroom will help towards a peaceful sleep.

Make sure your child goes to bed feeling loved, appreciated and safe. This may sound simple but they are basic human needs and extremely strong in children. To deny them causes huge emotional stress and will result in other health issues.

This first decade of your child's life is the one in which you will have the most influence; you are the centre of their world and they will still be looking to you for the answers to all life's questions. It is an enormous responsibility and one that if people thought about it too much most would probably never choose to become parents. But day by day we tip-toe our way through the minefield of parenting and with some guidance we can create a strong foundation in a child so they become a wonderful, inspirational, well-rounded and educated adult that can contribute to society positively and happily.

Modern-day society does not seem to fulfil this model, its morals appear lost and its social compass is in a flat spin but individual by individual and with love and determination, we can change the course of self-destruction that we are on and teach the next generation to do it better. You have ten years maybe 20 to do this vital job. Good luck!

CHAPTER 15

The Teenage Years!!!

One word......Hormones!!

Hormones are best viewed as a silent, deadly enemy - some alien being that has taken away your child and replaced it with a grumpy, screaming, emotional being that looks like your child but no longer acts like your child. They are actually performing a small miracle inside our children, they are cell by cell turning them into adults and although this process can seem endless, it is like everything in your journey as a parent - just another phase. As well as hormone changes, there are other new influences such as peer pressure, drugs, smoking, alcohol, learning to drive, sex and relationships, pressure from school and career choices to be made. It can seem overwhelming to a child that one minute was kicking a ball around with their friends at primary school and next not even understanding why they just reacted the way they did to a comment or action. It is confusing and complicated and it is a difficult phase for many. You will see all these mountains ahead of you and will most likely be panicked by how to navigate them all. The stress load on parents is enormous through this phase as the deep desire to keep your children safe is coupled with the understanding that you need to let them go and stretch their wings.

The best course through this phase is to create a solid grounding in healthy living as early as possible. If you have had the benefit of raising children with these values in earlier years, they will have formed habits that serve them really well as the challenges of teenage years loom. Without doubt, hormone levels fluctuate up and down, moods vary and tempers flare, emotions can be high and low with just minutes in between. It is only under the influence of powerful hormone changes that a child's body morphs into the new reality of an adult body. In my opinion, the best we can do to ease that transition is to create balance in areas we have control over. Areas such as diet, exercise, sleep, hobbies and daily routines.

Basic rules like ensuring children always have breakfast before leaving the house, having set bedtimes, yes even for teenagers, if they still live in your house you can set bedtimes. Sleep is where the body does most of its growth and repair, where it re-calibrates itself and it is extremely important that teenagers get the sleep they require. Their body clocks do change, they suddenly develop the ability to stay up later and the inability to get up early, this can be changed back by creating habits.

Limit screen times, especially in the evening; prioritise homework and jobs before any other activity. Involve children in shopping, cooking and cleaning up, you are not there to provide for their every need, you are there to teach them how to be independent human beings, ready to step out into the world and live independently and be self-sufficient. In a few short years they will be wanting to go and too many leave home ill-equipped to look after themselves.

I have written this book with the intention of covering the basic principles of living, showing you how to live a lifestyle to remove toxins and supply sufficiency for all our human needs. From pre-conceptive care to our last breath, so many of the principles remain the same so if you are reading this before you have children, you have years to set things up correctly for yourself and any children. However, you may have a teenager already and be looking for quick-fix solutions. If time is on your side, you can guide, cajole and teach for years and this is by far the simplest approach. Follow all the information you have read so far and introduce as much of it as you can and you will have a plain sail through those turbulent teenage years. It cannot be a coincidence that children and parents that live this way have a better experience through these teenage years, they live free of spots, no weight issues, no behavioural problems, no mood swings with no addictions or other health issues. I have had the absolute privilege of being mum to three amazing children, all now in their twenties, as soon as I learnt this information I actioned it and I feel pretty confident in saying that all three of the children would say it worked!

They have carried so many principles I have taught them into their adult lives, they all live independently now and I can say with conviction that they "own" the health information I have taught them. When I say taught, I did not sit down and teach them like school, instead we lived it all, we walked, we talked, we laughed, we played, we ate well, we treated illness with respect and allowed the body time to get well. They never reach for medication when ill, they reach for food that will support their bodies to get well and just give it time to work its magic.

Trust that the body works as a perfectly balanced machine until we interfere with its processes, then we stir up problems. If you want to have a happy, balanced teenager it starts by creating a happy, balanced body.

If you already have a teenager then you need to act fast and you need to lead. DO NOT expect them to change without changing yourself. You are their role model and even if they act as if they hate you, they still need you and they do take note of what you do. They are still learning even if they act as though they know it all and as long as you can give good reasons that stand up to their questions, they will respect you and not be able to argue against a new regime. Teenagers have some basic drivers, most want to be spot-free, slim, fit and socially accepted. Social media is giving them an impossible reality to live up to and that may need some very careful managing. We spend our entire childhoods trying to fit in and our adult lives trying to stand out, teenagers are in transition during this phase and often get it wrong but bear with them, they are learning on so many levels.

Behaviours are learnt, no one is born with a set of beliefs, we develop our own, therefore at any point we can rewrite what we think we believe and live a new reality. Our behaviours are dictated by our beliefs and our beliefs dictate our feelings about any given situation. You have to change the belief in order to change the feeling and then change the action and behaviour. It may sound complicated but it is actually very easy. If you give a teenager a new reality, a new belief they will be able to defend that position because they have new information and believe that. For example, it is a futile exercise to tell a teenager not to drink milk, firstly as the parent, you obviously know nothing and are just trying to manipulate them! However, if you can show them and explain to them the reasons why you are saying milk is not good for them, they will begin to accept that information and change their own belief system around the choice to drink milk. If they understand the process involved in milking cows, producing milk, the hormones and foreign cells in milk, the issues with digesting it, then they may choose not to drink it. At that point your work is done, they have changed their belief around something and they will actually go on and educate others. With information they will always been able to defend any position they hold on food or any other issue, my kids found this really,have tried very hard never to dictate what they must do, instead I have always tried to educate and allow them to make up their own minds. Life is about making constant choices and our compass for those decisions is our own belief system. Instilling the correct belief system is all it takes to have trust in your children's decisions.

I believe strongly that generation Y's and Z's , in the words of Peta Kelly in her book Earth is Hiring, have a divine intolerance to the world they are stepping into. They are living through the biggest change in millennia and they will be the generation that through education, passion and strong beliefs says, enough, there is a better way, our way. Watch us!

Before these amazing humans can grow up and change the world, they still have to course their way through these troublesome years. In reality, most children do not judge each other on what they are eating. Children that live a healthy lifestyle and diet are not excluded because they do not drink Coke; they are no less cool because they do not chew gum and if they choose not to binge-drink and smoke because they see that as a suicidal choice, then let them be judged on the fact they want to live, not die. Educated and informed children make the right choices, not because we as parents have laid down some rules with punishment. Instead, we give them information and explanation, we lead and act as role models and that is all that is needed. Luckily for us, good health feels great, so once you have that for yourself and you are role-modelling it for your children, once it is firmly ingrained as a lifestyle, it is actually a really hard thing to give up. Even teenagers prefer to feel well, have energy, look great, achieve well and sleep well.

Of course we all go off the rails sometimes but knowing how to get back on those rails is really important. That's what you can teach your children by modelling a healthy lifestyle.

So, exactly how are you going to navigate the teenage years? Luckily for us, a teenager can be treated as an adult as far as food choices are concerned, they have a few years to finish off their growth phase and their requirement for high quality nutrients through these years is enormous. This is not a need just for calories, it is a need for nutrition.

We need protein, carbohydrate and fat as well as micronutrients such as vitamins, minerals and enzymes. We need to be well hydrated with clean, pure water every day, and to eat fresh, raw natural food daily.

This on the surface seems like a nightmare request for a teenager living off junk food and fizzy pop, but a quick boost in the right direction soon has them looking and feeling better and able to embrace more of the changes. Remember, good health feels great and often the first obvious change is better skin - that alone inspires them to carry on.

The first rule is to add something good, do not just take something away. Removing things in phase one makes it seem hard, puts teenagers in rebellious mode and is almost always doomed to failure.

Your child will probably need reminding that as long as they live under your roof, they still need to comply with family decisions. When they are financially independent they can do things their way but until then, there are boundaries which need to be in place. Do not be scared to take this line, they should always respect you enough for this to be understood.

This next point is SO important - you absolutely must do whatever you are asking them to do. You need to be a role model. They will never change if you do not, so if you do not believe this is the course to improved health, then you will not be able to convince them.

You may have a very motivated teenager, in which case you will have an easy route to change or you may meet resistance and be unable to change them. Do not be too disappointed if this happens, all human beings have their own will and you cannot change someone who does not want to change, but you can educate. Over time they will find it harder and harder to argue against truth. Even teenagers cannot win that one. They can be stubborn and wrong but they only hurt themselves and when they see change around them that works, they start to feel a bit stupid for not following. They eventually come round, so just focus on the positive and change yourself and everyone in the family you can get to comply.

Top tips for teenagers

Take omega 3 daily

Take a probiotic daily

Drink 2 litres (4.5 pints) of water daily

Eat raw food – fruit or vegetable before each meal

If you can get your child to do these four things, even if they change nothing else, they will be helping their body function at a much improved level. This change can be undertaken without removing anything from the diet that may be toxic. This is a good bargaining tool for a reluctant teenager as you can bargain an addition and promise not to remove something they love. Remember no deprivation, at first all addition.

The next thing you need to add in is exercise, you need to get your teenager to agree to some daily activity. Discuss what they would enjoy, either a team or an individual sport, the actual activity does not matter but just like a young child, a teenager will only exercise if it is fun so work out what they find fun and make it part of their routine. Maybe this is something you can do with them and create an opportunity for building a more adult friendship. Many good parent/child relationships develop into adult friendships based around a common sporting interest.

If you have a motivated child that has a goal in mind, like weight loss or skin improvement, you can employ very particular strategies that show fast results and empower children to carry on.

Children should understand about food groups and nutrients and how their bodies are looking for particular foods to complete particular jobs within their bodies every day and if those things are not eaten, then they cannot complete the task. It is like trying to make a cake with no eggs!

Understanding food and why we need it?

Think of your body as a bank and your food intake as deposits you make within that bank. Withdrawing from the bank depletes your deposits but is necessary for survival so you must continue to make regular deposits in order not to go overdrawn.

Food is the starting point of the nutrient journey, everything we eat needs to be broken down and then rebuilt into what is required by the body. We are blueprinted within our DNA with what are in effect recipe books for every need the body has. Every part of our digestive system is perfectly designed for a particular job. However, we begin to run into some serious health issues when we either eat rubbish food with no nutrients for the body to extract or we fail to absorb the nutrients the foods contain. Either way, the body will fail to grow and repair and signs of illness will develop.

We run into one major problem with our modern day food - some of it did not exist when our recipe books were being written and as a basic rule of thumb if it was not around 40,000 years ago, our body has no idea what to do with it. Think of some modern-day food inventions like margarine and artificial sweeteners and then imagine the havoc those substances can create within the body when they is no recognition within us for them and no way to break them down or utilise them. There are many examples of "manmade" foods that the body literally has no idea what to do with!

Food represents the building blocks for life and if we fail to eat the foods we genetically require to be healthy, we will ultimately get sick.

Understanding Fats

Fats are necessary for –

Cell membrane integrity, omega 3 is required by every single cell in your body and you have 75-100 trillion cells!

For use as neurotransmitters, nerve message conduction relies on fats to relay their signals

In all steroid hormone production, that includes all reproductive hormones and stress hormones.

As a source of energy – they provide energy, the body's equivalent of rocket fuel

They provide the body with insulation and protective cushioning.

Essential fats for the body are Omega 3, 6 and 9 and cholesterol. No other fats are essential for the body.

Understanding Proteins

Proteins are made up of amino acids. There are 22 amino acids, eight of which are essential to human development and which the body is unable to synthesise and hence we have to include these in our food choices, otherwise we cannot build our own cells. All human tissue is made up of amino acids.

Understanding Carbohydrates

Carbohydrates consist of sugars and starches. The process of photosynthesis in plants produces starch which is our perfect carbohydrate food source. In a process using only water and sunlight, the plant produces glucose.

Sunlight + water + carbon dioxide = glucose + oxygen

This is the life-giving process that occurs on our planet and highlights the vital connection between plants and all life on this planet. They are our main source of energy.

Complex carbohydrates release their energy more slowly and help steady our blood sugars. They offer the best source of energy release and nutrient content. Examples of complex carbohydrates are whole foods where the food has not been broken down or processed. Imagine food as you would find it in nature, not processed and packaged.

Understanding Minerals

These are non-living substances found in nature that the body makes use of for various tissues and body functions

E.g. Calcium, iron, magnesium, phosphorus, sulphur, potassium, chlorine, sodium etc

Trace minerals are also essential such as iodine, copper, manganese, cobalt, nickel, zinc, chromium, selenium.

Minerals are drawn up out of healthy soil and held in suspension within a plant. These substances are fully accessible to us and are easily utilised by the body.

Understanding Vitamins

In nature, vitamins exist with co-factors. Without these co-factors the vitamins are rarely effective. This fact frustrates the scientist as he sits in his science lab trying to recreate the power locked in a fresh apple! He can reproduce a chemical copy of the vitamin but the co-factors are always missing.

Understanding Enzymes

Enzymes are protein-based agents that lend themselves to chemical reactions in the body. They remain unchanged by the reaction and can be used again and again. We have a finite quantity of enzymes that we inherit from our mothers. When we have used up all our enzymes we die! We can however obtain new enzymes from our food choices thereby replenishing our stock of them and prolonging our lives.

The most important fact to remember about enzymes is that they are destroyed completely above 40 degrees C.

They are used to aid every part of our digestion e.g. Lipase, amylase, lactase, peptase, protease, maltase etc are all enzymes used in every step of the digestive process.

If food is cooked you rely on your "bank account" of enzymes to break it down.

If your food is raw, you supply new enzymes with each mouthful.

Best sources of

- **Fats** - omega oils are found from animal sources, grass-fed meats and fish, especially oily fish and cold pressed, unheated plant oils. Whole grains offer a source of omega 6 but our intake of this should be carefully monitored as our current diets have most people's intake 20 times higher than it should be.

- **Proteins** – grass fed, non-hormone or antibiotic fed meat, dairy – the only acceptable source is raw milk that has not been pasteurised (nowadays almost impossible to obtain!), fish from non toxic seas, organic nuts, plants, grasses, algae and green, leafy vegetables, vegan protein with a full compliment of amino acids.

- **Carbohydrates** – without doubt the best source of these substances are plants. They offer complex carbohydrates in a perfect balance for our digestive system. They release their energy slowly and provide us with our most useable energy source. We can also gain some benefit from whole grains but remember that any split or processed grain will not be a beneficial form of energy for the body.

- **Vitamins** - due to the need for co-factors to be present, our only real viable source of vitamins comes from eating fresh, raw fruits and vegetables. Heating in any form destroys much of the vitamin content of the food and should be avoided as much as possible.

- **Minerals** – due to the fact that minerals come from the soil our only natural source of them is plant material. They are needed in minute amounts but are essential. Minerals do not require co-factors to work effectively, therefore man-made versions are more acceptable than chemically-produced vitamins.

- **Enzymes** – due to the fact that heat destroys ALL enzymes, there is no option but to eat raw fruit and vegetables to replenish your stock of essential enzymes. An amazing source of essential nutrients is wheatgrass, either taken as a fresh extracted juice or freeze dried powder it is a magic shot of all your enzyme requirements in one go. This extract cannot be recommended highly enough and is one that should be in a daily routine without fail.

Adding in Wheatgrass or Greens powder

This is the next goodie to put into your child's diet. One teaspoon per day in any juice will provide you with all your enzymes and amino acids each day. This is a real wonder food and an excellent short-cut to boosting up a system and for those reluctant vegetable eaters it is a good short-term solution. Ultimately, it is better to progress onto eating a variety of fresh foods but we can step our way into that, start by getting this superfood into them.

We all find it easy to be motivated to make changes born out of fear; kids love scary statistics but there is nothing much you can say to a teenager that will provoke enough fear to make them believe the choices they are making with their diet today will determine their future health and their predisposition to chronic illness. It is too much "in the future" for children to connect with but it is firmly understood now that our lifestyle choices affect our health. They feel invincible in these years and definitely do not live with the future in mind. Luckily, due to our phenomenal pace of regeneration in the first 20 years of our life, this pretty much goes un-noticed from the outside but internally your body has a long memory!

There are two things I will recommend that you stop straight away, the high sugar content of our foods and the continued use of artificial sweeteners, now proven to cause cancer, headaches, dizziness and mental deterioration to name but a few major issues. It is highly addictive and known to promote weight gain. It is prevalent in all diet foods, chewing gum, sweets, toothpaste, medications, (especially those for children!) fizzy drinks especially diet ones and many sweet foods.

A favourite argument from teenagers is "well they wouldn't sell it if it was dangerous!"

Oh YES they would!!!

Why would they not do so if they can make vast profits and hook in millions of people into an addictive substance that leaves you wanting more within hours?? These large companies DO NOT have your health as their motivating force, they only have their profit line and their commitment to their shareholders as their motivator.

Please do not ever get these things confused, if it is on shop shelves that is not a promise it is good for you, it is not even a guarantee that it is not bad for you - it just means the voices against its use have not managed to be heard yet against the enormous lobbies that can exist and the money that is thrown at legally shelving its ban.

Look back in history at times when this has happened both with foods and medications and do not believe it will not happen again. It will. You lose millions of brain cells with each mouthful of a diet soda, only you can decide if you think it is worth it.

Using high fructose corn syrup for extra sweetness has caused a pandemic of illness within the human species. Decisions made in the USA 40 years ago by farmers and businessmen trying to find a market for the cheap corn that was being produced in enormous quantities following the introduction of government subsidies for farmers, has now found its way into most of our manufactured food lines.

Monsanto, possibly one of the most powerful forces on earth as far as our food chain is concerned has had its fingers in the addictive sugar pie for decades. It has reaped the profits annually and refuses to address the health issues its products are causing; preferring to add more addictive ingredients rather than less to its foods and hooking more people in at a younger and younger age with the constant spread of its sugar-based products further and further into the market place.

To say that sugar wreaks havoc in our bodies is no exaggeration, it ages us, exhausts us, destroys our brain cells, clogs our arteries, confuses our hormones and along with cortisol and adrenaline (released when under stress) it is probably the single most important factor in the current pandemic of chronic illness in the human species. We are, without doubt, the sickest species on this planet, caused entirely by our own greed.

Changing the world view on this will take time, changing your personal decisions and that of your families can be done instantly. Becoming a conscious consumer is powerful beyond belief and as it spreads from person to person the world will change. Gram for gram there are theories that sugar does us more harm than heroin – a sobering thought when you think how many parents choose to give their children sugar in some form as a reward!

One large packet of jellied sweets contains on average 113 teaspoons of sugar! Just pause for a moment and think what your body has to do to process that, to register the soaring blood sugar levels, to pump out insulin at maximum output just to stop those spikes of blood sugar levels that can potentially kill us, the excess energy that hits our system, needing to be expended at just the same time the body needs to focus on controlling its biochemistry and saving our lives. There's the quick panic "store it until later" reaction that the body is forced to employ just to survive the onslaught and then the crash! Once the blood sugar levels are brought under control, the low that hits someone that has just had such an input of sugar is devastating. In every way it is a drug addiction and getting a teenager off sugar if they are hooked, is nothing less than removing their next fix.

Within two days, with good supportive nutrition, the chemical dependency is gone. The emotional connection to the sugar may take longer to break but with a strong will and an understanding of the damage it does, can also be easily overcome.

You do not need to ban all sugar forever, the human body works very effectively on sugar, it is a very important food source for us. However, knowing where to obtain healthy sugars is key - fruit sugars, vegetables, stevia, xylitol, agave nectar, natural honey, maple syrup, organic raw sugar and coconut sugar are all recognised by our brains, easily processed and can form a part of your diet. We function well on glucose; it is our main energy source. What we need to avoid are processed or artificial sugars and we need to respect the quantity of any type of sugar we ingest.

By a system of biochemical reactions within our bodies, excess sugar is converted into fat and stored.

It is not fat that makes us fat, it is carbohydrates and the prime culprit of carbohydrate foods that make us fat and cause all our chronic health issues is SUGAR!

Spots, weight issues, low energy, mood swings are all attributable to high sugar intake. If you want to make changes in any or all of those areas, cut the sugar out, the difference will be amazing.

There are so many areas I could highlight in how teenagers eat, move and think. Worryingly, our diets have never been worse, our exercise routines never poorer and our thought patterns are depressive and negative. Mental health issues are sky-rocketing, we are losing our sense of community, love and support. Many teenagers feel lost and scared, not supported or safe.

This sounds like a devastating picture and in some ways, it is. However, I believe that with education and guidance, this generation can embrace a new technology-based world and still be healthy. They need a guide to find the right path and a role model, they need to share what they've found and encourage others. The change is coming, we are literally on the cusp. We made a massive deviation away from good health in the seventies and we are paying a high price, however it has never been easier to access health products and a healthy lifestyle and the tide is truly turning.

There is an irony, I believe your teenager will most likely show you how to change some of your eating habits to save the planet, in my personal opinion, we should listen because if you've been living your adult life between the seventies and now, shame on us, we haven't done a very good job.

I wish you the best of luck creating friendships and adult relationships with your teenagers, this is as much about being a parent that is prepared to let go as it is about a child prepared to stay respectful and engaged with learning how to be an adult.

I have three of the most amazing humans in my life, I will always be mummy and yet these days I am also their friend. It is the most incredible journey to go on with a child and I hope for you and your teenager, you course a happy way to the other side of the parent-child relationship.

CHAPTER 16

How to Live a Complete Lifestyle and Create Wellness

As you have read through the different chapters of this book, I hope your eyes will have been opened to the simplicity of the changes needed and yet the enormity of the problem we have created. Understanding how we have become so sick as a species and giving you back control of your health destiny has been the mission of this book. You are just a few simple steps away from implementing all the changes you will ever need.

Before I conclude, let me recap on the basics. We develop chronic illnesses because we have toxicity and/or deficiency in three areas -

What we eat

How we move

What we think

Blowing apart old beliefs, the myths and sometimes the absolute lies we have been told, is all it takes to change a thought pattern and that will always lead to new behaviour.

The new behaviour will give you a new outcome to your health.

The behaviour is the action you will take, please do not think you can read this book and this new knowledge alone will propel you to good health. It is at this point you are required to take action.

The previous chapters have given you the background and new foundations to the way forward for you and your family. Now it is up to you!

You first need to find your "why"? your reason to go on this journey. Maybe you are driven by a fear of being ill, being dependent on others, being immobile, being in pain and will take action based on preventing that alone. Maybe you know what great health feels like and you choose that over suffering every time. Or maybe you have faced, or are facing, a diagnosis of chronic illness, of a modern-day disease, maybe you are fighting your way through every day in pain and suffering and trying to find a way to get well.

Maybe you just want the best life possible, maybe you are willing to make changes for your family's sake. A strong motive can be being a role model for your children, to teach them all you know and give them the knowledge they will need to make the best health choices in their lives.

You will "lean" on your motivation as you embark on these changes, you will need to stay strong, hold the line and each day make health choices that put you on the success curve for health and not the slippery slope to sickness.

The Complete Lifestyle plan created a community around the globe over the last 10 years, this is invaluable for support, encouragement and to find a place where likeminded people reside. Luckily for you, the health revolution is moving with huge momentum right now. It has never been easier to find healthy foods, visit health-conscious restaurants, find information on topics and communities of people to support you. All you have to do is choose your own tribe and choose health!

No one is here on the planet to tell you how to live your life, in this book you have read about a simple approach to combatting a massive issue, you have learnt how to ask more questions and, more importantly, the right questions. You have learnt how looking backwards to learn more about the way our ancestors lived, is actually the only route to moving forwards on a different, healthier path. Using the rules outlined in the book, by removing acidic foods, have primarily a plant-based diet, eating organic, grass-fed meats only, drinking clean, filtered water from glass bottles, treating your bowels with the respect they deserve and each day eating for health - not for cravings or addictions - will deliver you improved health

If you need some tracks to run on, the following chapter will outline the Complete Lifestyle plan. If you want to become part of the community, or be guided through a 30-Day Refresh Plan to improve your gut health, remove acidic, allergenic and addictive foods at the same time as providing your body with high-quality, nutritious foods, then simply follow me on Facebook and join one of our plans, they run monthly.

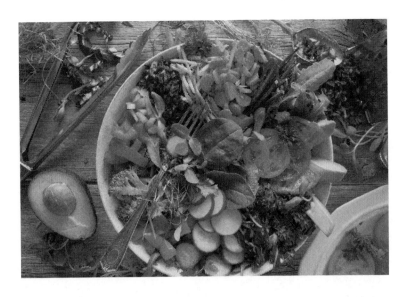

CHAPTER 17
Complete Lifestyle - 10 Step Plan

1. Eat fresh food, not manufactured products. Eat what nature provides in the form it is provided. Shop only from the edges of a supermarket where the fresh produce is and not from the inner aisles. Ask yourself if your great grandparents could have eaten it?? If not, maybe you shouldn't either!

2. Eat some raw vegetables or fruit with EVERY MEAL. They contain wonderful digestive enzymes as well as a multitude of other wonderful nutrients all in the perfect combination. Fruit in the morning and vegetables in the afternoon and evening is a good plan. The advent of smoothies makes this the simplest, yet most effective, health change you can make. Forget five a day, have 15 a day, all in one delicious drink! Heavy on the veg though!

3. Drink nothing other than clean water or herb teas. Do not drink water with your meal. This habit comes from eating processed foods that have no water content in them and not chewing your food properly. Take small bites and chew to a pulp before swallowing. There are no teeth in your stomach!

4. Slow-cook your lean, grass-fed meat and cook it thoroughly.

5. Pack homemade lunches - vegan protein shakes are wonderful and convenient for people on the go. Preparation is everything so you don't reach for the processed carb foods.

6. Get the right tools of the healthy eating trade. Get a slow cooker, a vegetable steamer, a juicer, a blender and some quality storage containers (preferably glass). Use stainless steel pots and pans not non-stick. If you are frying something, use organic heat tolerant oil such as avocado, coconut oil, sesame or almond oil for the non stick effect or some organic raw butter or ghee.

7. Enjoy your meals and eat small frequent meals rather than infrequent large meals. Food is supposed to be enjoyed and appreciated, however it is not supposed to be a source of emotional comfort or reward. There is a lot of talk currently about fasting, certainly giving your system a "rest" period from the onslaught of food is a good idea. A quick simple way to do this is to create a 12 hour window daily where no food goes in. This is easy to achieve when your window is between dinner and breakfast.

8. Don't ever shop hungry! The nutritional decisions that govern your health are made at the shops. If the "bad foods" come home, they'll get eaten. If they don't come home they can't get eaten and you will be healthier. Take

pride in going to the cashier with a trolley full of healthy foods for you and your family and take the opportunity to be an inspiration and leader for others. It's rare that the cashier doesn't comment on the amount of fruit and veg in my trolley at check-out and I feel a huge sense of pride every time they do!

9. Don't judge your dietary choices based on food guides, your neighbour's food, your parents' food, your workmate's food. Evaluate your choices on what you know your cells need to be healthy.

10. Never feel guilty about a food choice. Guilt will NEVER serve you well. Evaluate your food choices honestly but without personal character judgement. Always just look forward to your next meal as a chance to improve your eating habits and your health.

A Quick summary of Food Rules

- Eat some raw vegetable or fruit before every meal.
- Try and eat five meals a day, make breakfast and lunch your biggest meals.
- Chew your food thoroughly.
- Take Omega 3 (high quality molecularly distilled) and a probiotic daily (avoid yoghurt drink probiotics).
- Drink some fresh juiced vegetables from your own juicer every day.

   A vegan, protein - based smoothie is an amazing breakfast, packed with nutrients

- Eat only grass-fed, free-range, hormone-free meats.
- Make your own salad dressings.
- Limiting beverages other than water and herb tea to just once a day
- No dairy
- No artificial sweeteners
- No added salt
- No trans fats or hydrogenated fats
- Limit grains to one small serving per day if that is tolerated.

Treat days are fine, meals out are fine, just remember you have the ultimate control over your choices. Do not feel guilty though, the negative emotion of guilt is almost worse than the effect the food has. Be mindful of your mind and if you are going to have a treat ...enjoy it!

Try to never knowingly put toxins in your body, you are better to put "empty foods" in than toxic ones, for example if you fancy cake, make a cake, it will be an "empty" food nutritionally, except for calories, however a shop bought cake would give you a toxic load to deal with because it is packed with chemicals and other unnecessary ingredients.

Juicing - the power of liquid nutrients is incredible. Juices need to be predominantly vegetable-based as this has an alkalising affect on the body.

If you want to make life even simpler for yourself, a nutrient dense smoothie whizzed up in a NutriBullet delivers fibre, nutrients, enzymes and cofactors in a delicious drink. Start with 50% vegetables and top up with fruit, nuts, seeds and add in any power foods such as Acai, pea protein, goji berries, cacao, wheatgrass, spirulina etc etc.. It's hard to imagine a better start to anyone's day. If you are in the early stages of your health journey, this provides nutrition in an easily absorbable bioavailable way that allows your body time to rest from the process of digesting heavy foods. This rest phase then helps speed up the body's ability to let go of toxins. As we know, it's living toxin-free that helps us move up the health curve.

The 30-Day guided plan is based around nutrient-rich food being delivered in an easy-to-digest form, with supplements and meal choices that promote the release of toxins.

You may find yourself wanting to go on a health journey, yet surrounded by a family who don't share your excitement, the love of some of the recipes below usually wins everyone round and can be a way to get great nutrients into people that would say they hated fruit and veg!

The ingredients listed below in the recipes will be organic wherever possible, there are some top fruit and veg to ensure you always buy organic and others that are less important.

The Dirty Dozen - always buy these in organic form

Strawberries

Spinach

Nectarines

Potatoes

Apples

Grapes

Peaches

Cherries

Pears

Tomatoes

Celery

Sweet peppers

Go-To Favourite Juice!

3 apples

4 carrots

Large handful of spinach

1/2 lemon

1/2 cucumber

1/2 courgette

1/2 pepper

Chunk of ginger

1 inch slice of pineapple (skin on)

Optional extras include celery, broccoli, kale, beetroot or anything else that is lying around!

It's a good idea to put the spinach between the apples as you juice it.

Makes about a litre of juice.

Cleansing Juice

2 apples

1 small fresh beetroot

1 small stalk of broccoli

1/2 stick of celery

3 inch slice of cucumber

1 inch slice of pineapple

1 lime (peeled)

Optional extras can include a small handful of spinach or watercress and if you enjoy ginger as a flavour it is a nice addition

Calcium Rich Juice

2 apples

Handful of spinach

Chunk of broccoli

2 inch celery

Handful of kale

1 inch pineapple

3 carrots

1/2 lemon (rind removed)

Our greatest source of calcium are green, leafy vegetables and almost ALL fruits so if you make smoothies with real fruit, you'll be loading your system with calcium that gets straight to where it should be - your bones. But if you fancy using vegetables to get your calcium, then you'll need to juice them. I love the vegetables juiced with some fruit to sweeten the bitterness.

Orange Zinger

2 apples

chunk ginger

4 carrots

1 lemon (rind off)

1 orange (rind off)

If you want it to be sweeter, add a slice of pineapple through
the juicer

Berry Blast Smoothie

2 apples

Blackberries

Strawberries

Blueberries

(In fact any red berries you fancy)

Lemon or lime (rind off)

This is best as a smoothie, so blend, don't juice. This
can also be frozen to make the most amazing lollies.
This technique works brilliantly with fussy kids, make
frozen lollies out of nutrient-rich foods! If they won't
eat fruit or veg but love ice lollies. Parents, this is a
great way of getting those magic nutrients into your
children!

So, while I have just mentioned blending let me give
you a few of my favourite smoothies, made in a
blender not a juicer.

Cleansing Blast

1-2 handfuls of spinach

1 banana

1 cored apple

1 cored pear

1 cup of pineapple

Add water and whizz!

Immune Booster

1-2 handfuls of greens

1 banana

1 peeled orange

1 cup pineapple

1 handful of blueberries

Add water and whizz!

Life Booster

1-2 handfuls of kale

1 peach (stone removed)

1 banana

1 handful of strawberries

1/8 cup of flax seeds

1/8 cup goji berries

Add water and whizz!

Lastly, my absolute two favourites. For an added twist, add vegan protein

Chocolate Mint

2 scoops of vegan chocolate protein (I use Arbonne's)

Peppermint essence

Juice of 1/2 lime

Handful of spinach

Strawberries

Blueberries

Cashew nut butter (1 tbsp)

1/2 avocado

Whizz it all with water and serve chilled

Strawberry and Mango Delight

2 scoops of vegan vanilla protein

Handful of Strawberries

Handful of mango chunks

Juice of 1 lime

Add water and whizz!

These protein recipes also do really well as lollies!

This will just give you a flavour of the fun you can have with fruit and veg when juicing and blending and the nutrition that you can pile into each drink.

Juicers are easy to use, easy to clean, there is no chopping fruit and veg into small pieces anymore, just throw in whole fruits and veg and the machines do the rest. There are many on the market utilising different extraction techniques and depending on your health needs, you may be drawn to one over another. I do just encourage you to embrace this lifestyle and start to enjoy fresh, homemade juices.

The most popular blender available currently is the Nutribullet, it is simple, effective, affordable and offers everything you need. The power of the blender blades is the most important factor as that gives the smoothness to the drinks.

CHAPTER 18
Conclusion

I have struggled with knowing how exactly to finish off this book. The topic of health is so enormous and so diverse. The internet has placed every bit of information at your finger tips. I have been very mindful not to quote from scientific papers throughout this book because I can guarantee that whatever I write will become old news very quickly, yet the principles of health will remain the same.

If you are interested in the science of nutrition or disease, then I encourage you to delve deep into the topic and swim around in the information for a while. Allow yourself to percolate on the different ideas and see what fits with you, where does your truth lie? When you find your truth and know your belief system on health, so much of what you see and hear can be filtered out.

If you are interested in my daily routine for healthy living, it is trained out on the 30-Day plan and anyone is welcome to join that plan any time. I could have packed the last few chapters of this book with recipes and meal plans for an A-Z guide to living to prevent disease, however I feel that if you have truly read this book, you will understand how we are making ourselves ill, you will be able to identify where your personal stress load lies and it is from that point that you can start to change.

Chronic illness takes decades to create. Remember, if you are currently free of a diagnosis of a chronic modern-day illness, you have time. Start today and make the necessary steps to "Get Off Your Iceberg"

If you are living with chronic illness, your action needs to be harder and faster. Be intentional with every choice you make in your life; you need to eat for health, move for health and your mindset needs to be positive and stress-free.

Your personal stress load is like a carrying a rucksack around filled with stones, when the load becomes too heavy you cannot move. You can choose at any point in time to lift those stones out and leave them on the ground. After all you put them in there in the first place.

Health, good or bad, is a choice. You have sole responsibility for your own health. There is no blame that you can leave at the door of a manufacturer, a drug company, a doctor, your boss, your family etc The choice is always 100% yours, I encourage you to always ask one more question than you have the answer to and keep digging and asking until you have complete satisfaction on the answer.

To give you a simple example, imagine you are 60 years old, you have lived a stressful life in a job you haven't loved but you have tolerated. It has placed you at a desk or behind the wheel of your car for at least eight hours a day for the last 40 years. You eat on the run most days and live for your holidays and weekends. You have high blood pressure and are showing signs of developing diabetes. A doctor would tell you exactly what they have in front of them - a person with high blood pressure and pre-diabetes and they will tell you you need a drug to lower your blood pressure and they will monitor your bloods for sugar levels. Unless you personally ask WHY?, you will not be given that answer.

I hope as you read that you are screaming at the page "Get off Your Iceberg!!"

The route back to health is NOT a drug, it is a lifestyle change.

A drug will take the blood pressure down but if you stay in the same environment, you will push that pressure up again. The body is responding correctly, you are interfering with a good response by medicating. The pressure is only high because of the lifestyle choices -change the lifestyle and the blood pressure will lower - danger over, stress decreased, symptoms will disappear. It sounds so simple in theory and in many ways it is, however chronic illness can be life-threatening and serious so there are times that medical intervention is essential, (remember the fire brigade analogy) and saves lives. However, and I am shouting this with love at you, unless you get off your iceberg you will continue to get more ill, even if the symptoms are masked with medication!

Stop!!! Reassess your life, take some of those stones out of your back pack and start moving forwards with a lighter stress load.

The reason I have chosen not to give you the step-by-step guide is that many approaches work. You may fancy going plant-based in your diet, that may make perfect sense to you. You may decide to fast periodically, you may choose to be carb-free, dairy-free, wheat- free, you may juice daily, join a yoga class, run a marathon, leave your job, get into therapy, read self-help books, create a group or community yourself, you may move house, even countries, take a trip you always wanted to, you may research a topic and help others, you may develop a social media presence and educate others, you may write a book. I am not here to tell you one diet or lifestyle choice is better than the other, the point of this book is to show you we are getting it wrong right now. As chronic illness soars, we cannot in all logical consciousness continue to do the same thing.

We are creating an environment where an entire species is getting sicker and sicker and one of the things that truly saddens me is we are affecting many other species along our self destructive path.

It's time to wake-up, look at the evidence and take back the power; to work with, not against the miracle that is the human body; to educate and inspire people even if it is one person at a time to take back that control.

All actions have consequences and as long as you are happy with your own consequences, then your actions will be right for you. If, however, you feel you may be on the wrong path and you are not keen on the results you are heading for, then change your actions. Get off Your Iceberg!

Only you can choose to stand up, and walk away from that cold, uninhabitable iceberg, the one that is killing you one degree at a time.

Stand up and start walking in a new direction, it will save your life!

SUCCESS STORIES

How I Dropped Two Dress Sizes with Complete Lifestyle

As a 46-year-old, full-time working mum. I found it hard to fit any exercise into my busy day let alone think up fancy, low-fat recipes that would satisfy three hungry men back home.

Complete Lifestyle helped me change my habits gradually. The changes might have been subtle but the effect it had on my waistline was dramatic.

It all started when I was recommended to try a juicing programme for my son to ease sinus congestion. I thought I'd try it myself before giving it to him so turned to Complete Lifestyle for advice on introducing juices to my diet and making other simple changes to the way I lived my life.

After four days, I felt so good and had lost lots of weight so I decided to keep going having juices during the day and a meal in the evening.

Although it wasn't easy working full-time, juicing, exercising and running a house; I noticed the difference to my energy levels and my waistline very quickly. I also found the Complete Lifestyle programme offered great ongoing support to keep me motivated.

I've lost two stones and have inspired the whole family to eat healthily. Even my son Ben has started taking a piece of fruit to school instead of a chocolate biscuit. Wayne, my husband, has stopped his desserts and started running and my other son Tom is getting his head round juicing.

It's been a major lifestyle change but we've done it gradually and with plenty of support from Complete Lifestyle.

Debs, mum of two, aged 46

How One Man Beat Middle Aged Spread

Not many men my age will admit to going on a diet but plenty of us would secretly like to. In my case, I was almost two stones above my ideal weight and didn't like the way I looked. I didn't look good in the pool on holiday with the kids and I certainly didn't enjoy looking at myself in the mirror.

I decided to follow the Complete Lifestyle programme because it claimed that it wouldn't make me give up the things I enjoyed. That was certainly true. Once you try it, you'll realise that the subtle changes you make to the way you live mean you don't crave the foods you used to and you naturally opt for healthier choices.

As a business owner, I work long days, often 12 hours with little opportunity for a break. I started taking shakes to work to sustain me through the hectic days and cut down on sugary snacks.

As part of the programme, I chose to follow Complete Lifestyle's seven-day detox to accelerate my weight loss. On day one I weighed in at 97.8kg and at the end of the week I was down to 94.4kg.

I also started walking for an hour before work and took protein shakes in airtight flasks. My nightcaps changed from wine to peppermint tea and I not only dropped pounds, I also slept better than I had for a long time.

I am really pleased with my weight loss and will definitely continue to live a healthier lifestyle. I have loved adding good stuff in and now don't even feel like I want the bad stuff back.

Nigel, company director

Healthy Living for Body Conscious Teenagers

All people my age are conscious of the way they look but most teens also put all the wrong things into their bodies. In my case, I wanted to lose a little bit of weight, look more toned and get rid of my spots. I loved sweet things so I thought I would try and train myself to prefer other things.

I really enjoyed finding out more about which foods are good for you and which ones aren't. That information has really made me think about my diet.

It's hard to eat healthily as a teenager because you eat what everyone around you eats. My friends questioned what I was doing when I started choosing salads and fresh juices and protein smoothies instead of the usual snack foods but once I realised how good these things were making me feel, I didn't mind.

Matt, 15

I'd Tried Everything to Overcome My Son's ADHD

Having a child with special needs is not easy. Over the years, my son had been given many different labels.

Four years ago, ADHD was the label of the moment and as any concerned parent would, I sought to find anything that I felt could help with his symptoms.

I'm very open to alternative therapies and tried him with Reiki, EFT and Homeopathy to name just a few. I had pretty much come to a dead end and really didn't know where to turn.

An assessment from a chiropractor revealed that my son didn't have ADHD and the clinic introduced me to the Complete Lifestyle programme to run alongside the treatment being offered by the chiropractor.

Gradually, I discovered the positive impact on my son's body as I removed toxins like dairy, wheat and aspartame and added Omega 3, Acidophilus and lots and lots of fresh fruits and veg.

My son's school started to notice a difference in his behaviour and soon so did most people that knew him.

One day, I suddenly realised that while I had been making sure that he had been getting all these great things in his diet, I had totally neglected myself and not even taken into consideration that I would also benefit from all this stuff.

Wellness isn't just about what you're putting into your body, it's also about moving and thinking your way to better health. You look at your values and it's great when you start to think in a positive way.

Linda, 42

Complete Lifestyle Cured my Children's Asthma and Eczema

After a very pleasant but over indulged Christmas and New Year, I felt that something in our family nutrition had to be stepped up a little.

I have always been very health conscious but since having the three children we had got into a habit of lots of bread, dairy and what we call in our family "beige food".

I discovered Complete Lifestyle and became totally hooked and inspired.

My youngest daughter Phoebe has struggled with a wheezy chest and cough ever since she came into the world and after juicing carrot, apple, lemon and pineapple together with omega 3 oil every morning, I could see that it was such an easy way of increasing her daily vitamins naturally and helping to support her immune system. However, in March, she was hospitalised due to an asthma attack and was kept in for four days. Naturally as her mother, this was terrifying and I wanted to start looking at her diet more closely.

I followed Complete Lifestyle's advice to take the dairy and wheat out of her diet. I replaced cow's milk with rice milk and other plant-based milks. I can't tell you how much better her chest is and she's lost her cough altogether. Phoebe's twin brother, Peter, also struggled with eczema and this has now totally disappeared.

We have been following Complete Lifestyle for six months now, heeding advice to increase water intake, take omega 3, exercise regularly and decrease stress levels. The difference we feel is amazing. Our eldest daughter, Hannah who is four, has had nowhere near as many colds as last year. Her energy and concentration levels have increased tenfold and she has embraced her new eating habits. My husband was quite reluctant at the beginning and now he cannot get enough of it all, and you'll find him hovering in the kitchen waiting for his juice and protein smoothie every morning!

Lou, mum of three

Tess's Story

For all my life, I have been extremely fit and active. I never suffered with aches and pains or back problems until two years ago. I remember taking my Ma out to lunch for her birthday, I felt fine but suddenly during the meal I lost my voice. The next day, I felt really unwell and took to my bed. This lasted for a week and gradually I returned to normal - only to go down with the same virus a couple of weeks later. This happened three times in a very short period, each time the symptoms grew progressively worse. My body was racked with pain, all the strength had left my arms. I was suffering with chronic fatigue and it was now impossible to get out of a chair without immense willpower. I kept putting off going to the doctor, but eventually as the pain was taking me over, I decided to book in with my GP.

After blood tests and a visit to the rheumatoid arthritis consultant, I was told I had Polymyalgia (an inflammatory disorder that causes muscle pain and stiffness), my doctor rang me and said it was easy to cure, I would start off on a high dose of steroids and gradually reduce them..... that was like a red rag to a bull, I knew there and then that there was no way I was going to take steroids. So, having told the doctor I would go and see her the next day. Knowing I was not going to go, I decided I had to cure myself.

I decided to adopt a raw food diet. I am convinced when times are tough, you are guided and this was what was happening to me.

I decided I had to read and equip myself with as much knowledge as I could. I joined classes, visited experts (both in the UK and New York). The defining moment came when Denise who runs a clinic in New York told me: "You don't catch viruses!" But I had just caught three, one after the other. It was then she taught me about your inner terrain. If you are in an alkaline state, there is no way viruses and diseases can survive. However, if your body is in an acid state, which obviously mine was, then it is the prime condition for you to become sick. Wow! And there was I thinking I was eating a healthy diet. I also learnt that there are four main reasons why we become sick. 1. There are too many toxins in the body 2. There are nutritional deficiencies 3. Exposure to electromagnetic chaos 4. Stress.

I started to juice every day, eat salads and protein smoothies. The more raw I ate, the better my body felt. I could actually feel the nutrients seeping back into my body. I learnt from another raw food teacher about the importance of drinking one-and-a-half litres of green juice every day. I found it fascinating and I was loving my food. I learnt about live foods, dead foods, the importance of enzymes. I just felt everything was falling into place, for the first time in my life, I was actually understanding food.

Big problems arose with my friends - they were horrified that I was eating like this and also refusing painkillers or medication, At first, I felt embarrassed telling them but once I could feel the difference in my body, I decided to ignore the comments.

As the months passed I could see and feel amazing changes in my body. I was having Rolfing massage every week, to help ease the pain, I was sticking with my raw food and juicing. Gradually, I started to feel normal again. It has taken me about 18 months to feel totally cured, but I knew it wasn't going to be a quick fix.

Today, looking back on my journey, I feel really privileged that I was ill, which seems a very strange thing to say, but I now really understand why we get sick and how we can cure ourselves without resorting to prescriptive or over-the-counter drugs and surgery.

My friends who initially thought I was completely away with the fairies, are now coming to my classes and investing in vita-mixes, NutriBullets and juicers. They see the changes in me and want to know what I'm up to.

I have invested huge amounts both in time and money to educate myself, and I now feel passionate about helping others take responsibility for their own health. I truly believe you can only be healthy when you take responsibility for yourself, no pill, doctor or friend can cure you of disease, only your own understanding and body can do that.

Linda's Story

Shingles Schmingles!

If you've ever had shingles, you will appreciate what I'm saying when I say the pain in my side was unbearable - and I consider myself to have a high pain threshold. I wouldn't wish it upon anyone.

What I would advise you to do is to visit a chiropractor..... yes really a chiropractor. Having spent a few days in pain, I went to see my wellness chiropractor Debbie (who diagnosed my shingles). She explained that I needed to get lots and lots of good things into my body, your body heals and is well from the inside out. So, I started taking one teaspoon of wheatgrass every morning and really stepped up my daily juicing regime, ensuring that I had lots of green juices, spinach, kale, avocado & lime were all particular favourites. I was adjusted once a week at the clinic and Debbie encouraged me throughout the process. I continued to work and have a normal life, despite the fact that when I had told other people what I had, they had said things like:

"Oh you'll be off work for weeks with that, maybe even months."

Or "When I had that I was in bed all day."

Or "I had shingles years ago and I've never really got over it!"

Despite these, and other comments, I stayed positive and I knew that by following the guidance from Debbie, I would be well, I would recover and that I would not feel the ill-effects of shingles for years to come.

Three weeks later and having done all that I have said, I can say that my shingles was well and truly banished, I'm still keeping up with the wheatgrass and the juicing, I have treats just the same, however I know that by adding in good things, I am giving my body the right fuel for a healthy and happy life.

Linda, 42

Helen's Story

Ok. Bit of an update from me. This is a long post so please read to the end. For those who have come over from the June page, you know my story. For those who are only on day 2 of this diet (I know, I know, it's a detox lol) and maybe struggling with lack of coffee and having a headache etc I will explain and hopefully inspire you to continue. I am a breast cancer survivor. I like writing that. Chemotherapy, whilst doing me the enormous favour of killing the cells that tried to kill me, also diminished (probably for ever) my ability to heal. For six and a half years I have battled infection after infection and had the unpleasant side effect of two substantial holes in my left boobatron, which simply would not heal. Suffice to say I would have to change my bedding twice weekly as these open, weeping sores would make a mess on my sheets. Anyway, the last stage in my cancer journey and hopefully the last of my 15 operations thus far is to have my new nipple tattooed. A little over a month ago I was back at the hospital to see my 3B surgeon. I call him 3B because he is big, black and very, very beautiful. He was concerned about my wounds. I couldn't possibly tattoo while there was such infection, not to mention the open sores. He took a swab. Ten days into my diet (I know, I know...) miraculously the wounds healed. Six and a half years of waiting and all I really needed to do was eat clean. So, that's where we were until today. I am currently in the multi-storey at the hospital weeping tears of joy. Wearing my best bra for my beautiful 3B, he could not believe his eyes (haha - have had this effect on so many men whilst in my bra lol). He even stuttered. 'B-b-but I was going to tell you that the results of your swab suggested that we wouldn't be able to go ahead. There was massive infection. What have you done different?' I explained about Clean and Lean. He was amazed. And above all else, he has given me a date. Not that sort of date - I'm a married woman. But a date for my tattoo. A date for this hideous, nearly seven year journey to be over. Debbie Townsend I can't thank you enough. This would NEVER have happened without Arbonne. Plus as I left his consulting room he said 'You've lost weight, too!' BOOM. X

Alona's Story

My name is Alona, I am 46 years old, I have a 27-year-old son, I am a teacher and I have been seeing Debbie since (I can't remember).

Initially, I came to see a chiropractor for help because for years I thought that I suffered with sciatica nerve in my lower my back and in the back of my legs. At times, the pain was unbearable and I survived on strong painkillers and by soldiering through.

I was amazed; the relief didn't come immediately, but gradually, session after session my spine was stronger, my pain has lessened, I could ditch those painkillers and manage the pain. Every time I came for a treatment, Debs would give me an advice on how to manage my lifestyle in order to remain healthy and minimise that excruciating back pain.

She then introduced me to the first edition of Complete Lifestyle, where she described and gave examples of how to live a simple, affordable and healthy lifestyle. Personally, my favourites were: any advice about diary and how the species with the most healthy skeletal system i.e elephants and gorillas don't consume any dairy at all, other than mother's milk when they are infants.

The second one came from an advice to ditch sugar replacements, such as sweeteners etc.

I followed her guidelines and can honestly say, that I have never looked back. I eat very healthily, I exercise twice per week, I don't walk as often as I should but I can confidently say that those little bits of advice have helped me massively to improve my lifestyle.

Alona, 46

Maureen's Story

Four weeks ago, all my joints muscles ached, hurt, I was dragging myself up the stairs, my legs felt like dead weight, I had no energy and was so tired. Discovering my skeletal system was inflamed, I was advised to try the 30-Day to Healthy Living programme. After four weeks, the aches and pains had gone! No more pulling myself up the stairs, I'm running up now, energy back. I'm actually sleeping better, after years of not.

The icing on the cake - I have lost 6lbs in weight and a couple of inches off my waist!!!! A big thank you to Debbie, without her introducing me to this plan, I would not feel like I do now.

I will definitely continue with healthy, clean cooking, without a doubt. I have learnt so much, not really missed a lot, but will gradually put back certain foods as suggested. But not a lot.

Thank-you so very much for encouraging me to do 30-Day plan, best thing I've done, so pleased!

And now knowing the results, I can dip back into it whenever I need to. No more pain!

Maureen, 56

Holly's battle against Fibromyalgia

Hello, my name is Holly and I want share my experiences with some healthy lifestyle changes and how it has impacted me and my family.

I am a single, working mum of two beautiful children (aged 6 and 9) I was diagnosed with Fibromyalgia in June 2017. At the time I was shocked, I knew I'd had a few rough years, a surprise pregnancy, a child that never slept, a stressful job safeguarding children, a split with the children's father, and so I had put my symptoms down to life and not a chronic illness.

Looking back now, I am unsure how I managed. I suffered migraines three or four times a week, I felt bloated all the time and had IBS. I was dragging myself out of bed after more than eight hours sleep, still exhausted, I had lots of nightmares, my limbs ached all over, I was unable to concentrate and started to forget things, I stuttered as I couldn't process the words in my head. My head felt like it was in a spaceman's helmet and I knew it was impacting my work. I was grumpy, snappy and I'll admit it, not a great mum or person to be around.

The symptom that left me the most devastated was the pain and lack of strength in my hands, unable to tie my daughters hair up or do the children's buttons on their clothes. All this left me demotivated and low in mood.

The doctors told me there was no cure, fibro had only recently being recognised as a chronic illness and it was in its early stages of research. I'd have to prepare myself to be unable to continue working, the illness will only progress and get worse. I was prescribed lots of pain killers, muscle relaxants and anti depressants to mask the pain.

I refused to accept that this would be my new reality, so I decided to write a new ending to my book of life.

I started to research the healthy benefits of nutrition. There was so much to unravel, it seemed like a minefield. There was such a lot of research out there, some of it was conflicting, differing information dependent on what you wanted the outcome to be. I was completely confused and overwhelmed. I tried some of the suggestions on offer, some worked initially but nothing seemed to be sustainable and after a while I was back to square one.

I was then introduced to a healthy eating plan by Debbie. This program pulled together everything I had been researching, into an easy-to-follow plan. The recipes were straightforward and looked simple to cook for this novice chef who also had a family to feed.

But would it have an impact on my health? Would plants be better than prescribed medication?

For the first time, I was not restricting my body from gorgeous foods, I was replacing the foods that didn't serve my body for ones that did. I made small changes to my diet and how I cooked. Over time, this changed my mindset around food. And I loved it. After a shaky start, the kids are wolfing the food down and asking for seconds. My biggest battle was getting rid of dairy, which I've finally done thanks to some fab alternatives and recipes the children think are treats.

Within days, my migraines had gone. I was surprised that I'd made such small changes for such a massive impact and it only got better. I found I was sleeping without nightmares and waking refreshed and was more focused throughout the day. I felt like a fog had been lifted from around my head and my thoughts were being formed into words and flowing out of my mouth easily. I lost weight, felt less bloated and that uncomfortable feeling after eating disappeared.

After the second month of continuing the plan, the pains in my hands had reduced so much that I was able to help the children thread needles and sew handmade Christmas decorations - something I would have never been able to even attempt the Christmas before.

I feel empowered in the knowledge that I have so much control over my health and have in my hands a really simple plan I can follow. The plan helps me understand what I can do to fully support my body, so that it can work at its best. I can't believe how easy it was to make the changes. I stopped listening to all the stories in my head "I cant do this because..." and just started trying. I've made mistakes along the way, at times its felt like two steps forward, one step back. But I've learnt from those mistakes, which is what mistakes are for after all and I am moving forward, happy in my healthy living lifestyle.

Holly, 36

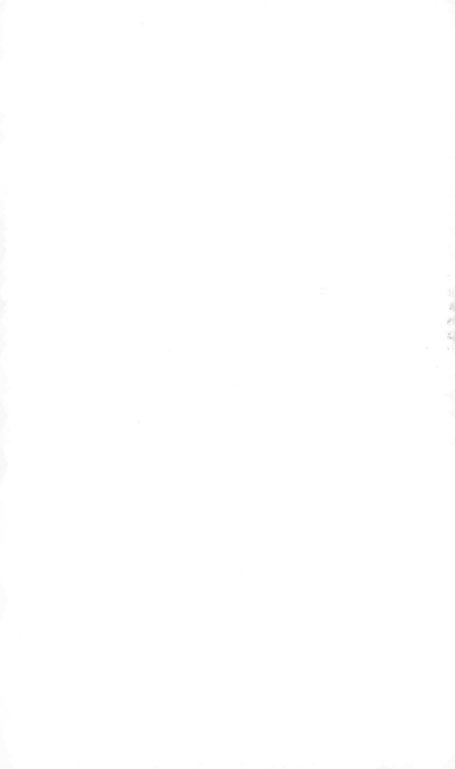

Printed in Poland
by Amazon Fulfillment
Poland Sp. z o.o., Wrocław